Pharmacology

Crossword Challenge

Perspectives, Medication Calculations, Pharmacology Issues, Autonomic Nervous System, Neurologic & Neuromuscular Agents, Pain & Inflammation, Psychiatric Agents, Antibacterial Agents, Immunologic Agents, Antineoplastic Agents, Respiratory, Cardiovascular, Gastrointestinal, Eye, Ear & Skin, Endocrine, Reproductive, Emergency Agents and Glossary

Medpuzzles, LLC

www.Medpuzzles.com

Pharmacology
Crossword Challenge
Perspectives
Drug Administration & Principles
Section I

Across

3. According to the Joint Commission, this is not an acceptable abbreviation for ordering or documenting medications.
6. The act of drawing in the breath, drawing a medicated agent with the breath; a solution of a drug or combination of drugs for administration as a nebulized mist intended to reach the respiratory tree
7. This term is used to describe a corner of the eye.
9. This category of drug orders may be an ongoing order given for a specific number of doses or days or may have a special instruction to base administration on laboratory values.
11. Do not use this in site; IM injection in children.
13. An advantage of the unit dose method of drug distribution is increased _____ l
16. These agents are examples of autonomic drops.
18. A commonly used abbreviation include: gonagiluteal, dalteid; vastus lateralis and ____
19. The typical sites for IM injections should be read ____ times.
21. To avoid drug error the drug label should be read ____ times.
23. The tearing in incorporation, or reception of gases, liquids, light or heat.
24. Pull down and back on the auricle when administering ear drops to ____
26. The pattern of occurrence of a substance within or between cells, tissues, organisms
27. A technique to estimate the amount of medication remaining in a canister is to place the canister in ____
28. The preferred site for a medication ordered via the IM route for a 9-month old child is the vastus ____

Down

1. The First-Four-Five Rights: include the right: Client, drug, dose, assessment and ____
2. This term describes a bitter or a bleb
4. HCT is an example of an ophthalmic that is ____
6. Needles should ____ be recapped
8. The main route of drug excretion is via the ____
9. This route of administration involves placing the drug under the tongue for venous absorption.
10. This effect occurs when the drug is metabolized or excreted more slowly than the rate at which it is being administered.
12. These are devices used to enhance the delivery of medications from metered-dose inhalers
14. This is the name of the route used when placing the drug between the gum and the cheek
17. Because IM administration is painful and may cause tissue irritation, this broad spectrum antibiotic is typically administered orally or IV.
18. This is at the time of the desired dose
20. A type of medication administration whereby the drug was placed directly onto the skin
21. This term refers to the first adverse symptoms that
22. A box or container
25. This method of drug distribution includes drugs

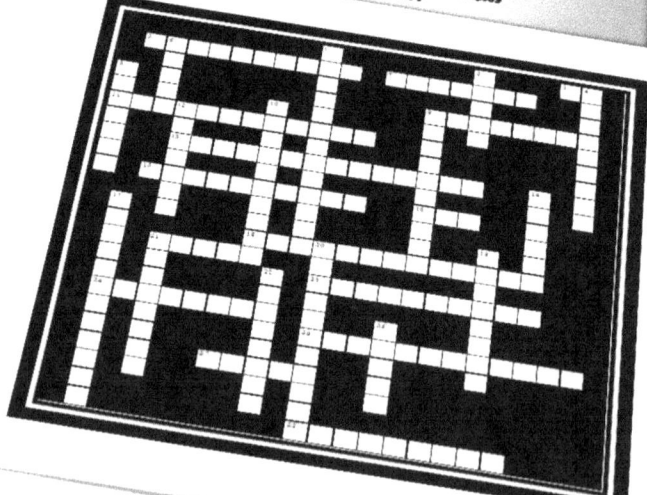

Pharmacology
Crossword Challenge
Perspectives
Drug Administration & Principles
Section I

Patricia O'Brien-Giglia, CMT, began her career in the healthcare field after having graduated from The Broward County Practical Nursing Program in 1980 to achieve her LPN license. She continued her education by graduating with her Associate in Arts degree from Seminole Community College in 1993.

Having served on the Editorial Advisory Board as an editorial consultant for Stedman's (Lippincott Williams & Wilkins), she has participated in the completion of *Radiology Words, Fourth & Fifth Editions,* as well as having developed crossword puzzles accompanying CD for Lippincott Williams & Wilkins' *Medical Terminology Quick & Concise, A Programmed Leaning Approach.* Patricia has contributed to and has been acknowledged for her contributions toward *The Medical Transcriptionist's Guide to Microsoft Word, Third Edition, Make It Your Own.*

Patricia currently resides in Tampa, Florida employed as a Medical Transcription Supervisor for a major cancer center where she developed their Medical Transcription Department Quality Assurance Program.

Currently enrolled in The University of South Florida, she is working on her BSAS in Public Health.

She is a member of the Audubon Society, enjoys photography and gardening and continues to keep her website www.Medpuzzles.com up to date for all of her students and teachers in the healthcare field.

Pharmacology
Crossword Challenge
Table of Contents

Pharmacology
Crossword Challenge
Table of Contents

Across

4. A psychologic benefit from a compound without the chemical structure of a drug effect is known as a ___ effect.
5. The first phase of drug action.
6. This type of reaction is more severe than side effects.
8. This lab test is the most accurate way to determine renal function: ___ clearance.
11. This drug is an example of a moderately highly protein-bound drug.
12. Drugs given by this route involve only pharmacokinetic and pharmacodynamic phases.
15. The process by which a drug becomes available to body fluids and tissues.
16. These types of food decrease absorption rate.
17. This type of absorption occurs mostly by diffusion.
18. The main route of drug elimination is through ___.
21. A subcategory of absorption, the percentage of administered drug dose that reaches systemic circulation.
24. The time it takes to reach the minimum effective concentration after a drug is administered, the ___ of action.
25. This drug is an example of a low protein-bound drug.
26. Drugs are disintegrated and absorbed faster in ___ acids
28. The highest plasma concentration of a drug at a specific time.
29. This term describes fillers and inert substances used in drug preparation.
32. An example of a drug that is highly protein-bound.
33. When a drug has a low therapeutic index, it is considered a ___ margin of safety.
34. A large initial dose given when immediate drug response is desired.
35. Protein-bound drugs cannot be filtered through the ___.
36. Drug distribution is influenced by blood flow, the drug's affinity to the tissue and the ___binding effect.

Down

1. Penicillin is poorly absorbed by the GI tract because of ___acid.
2. Another term for biotransformation is called ___.
3. The breakdown of a tablet into smaller particles.
4. This phase is the study of drug concentration and its effects on the body.
7. An example of a drug that is low protein-bound.
9. Four sequential processes of pharmacokinetics: Absorption, distribution, metabolism and ___.
10. This organ is the primary site of metabolism.
13. Rapid decrease in response to a drug.
14. The movement of drug particles from the GI tract to body fluids by passive absorption.
15. A tablet undergoes disintegration and ___ before it is absorbed.
19. A drug that is 75% protein-bound is classified as ___highly protein-bound.
20. This drug is an example of a first-pass effect drug.
22. The process in which a drug passes to the liver first is called first-pass effect, or ___ first pass.
23. Decreased responsiveness over a course of therapy.
27. A decrease in liver function can ___the bioavailability of a drug.
30. The lowest plasma concentration of a drug, drawn before next dose is given.
31. This form of a drug is absorbed faster than solid.

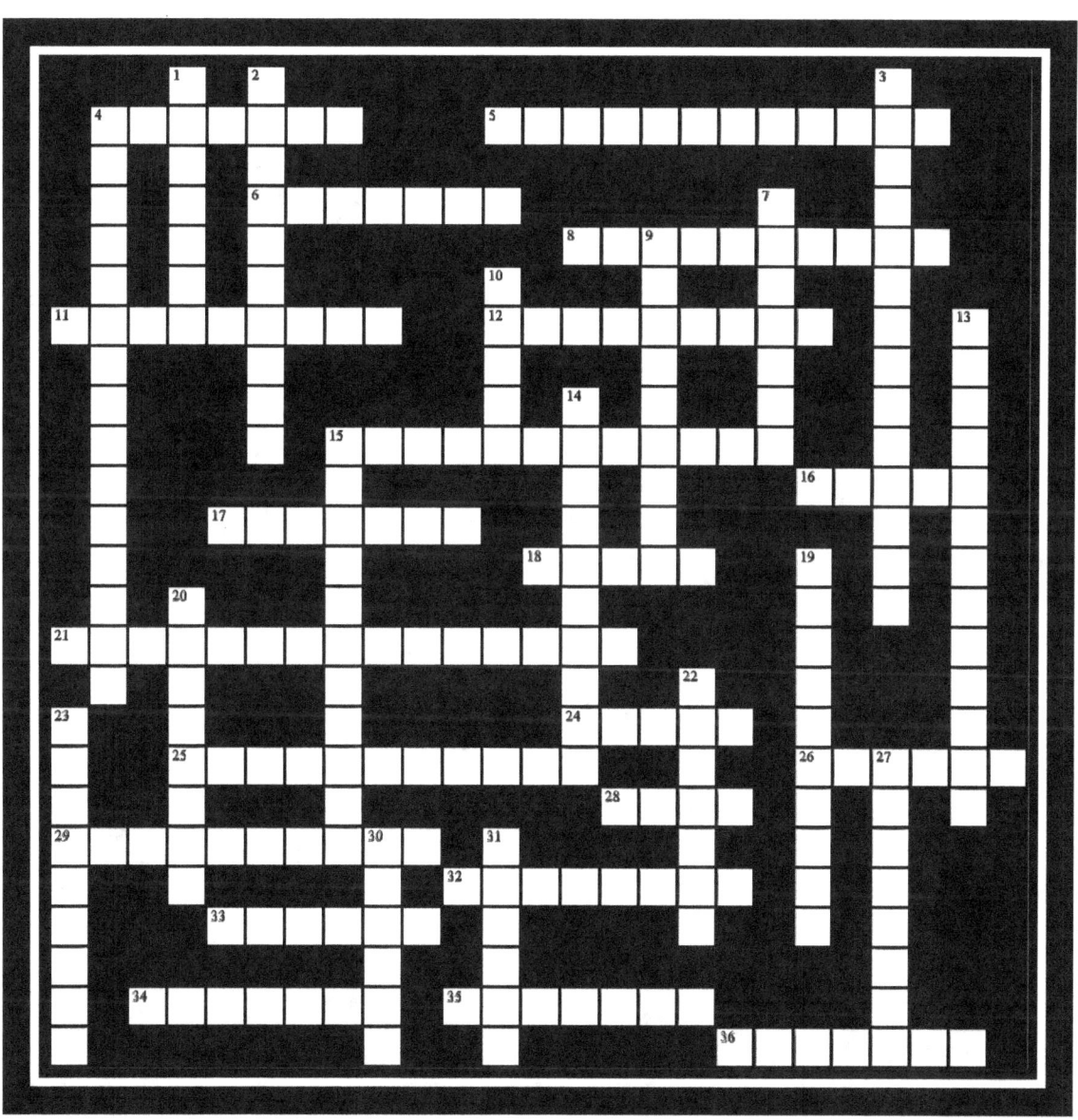

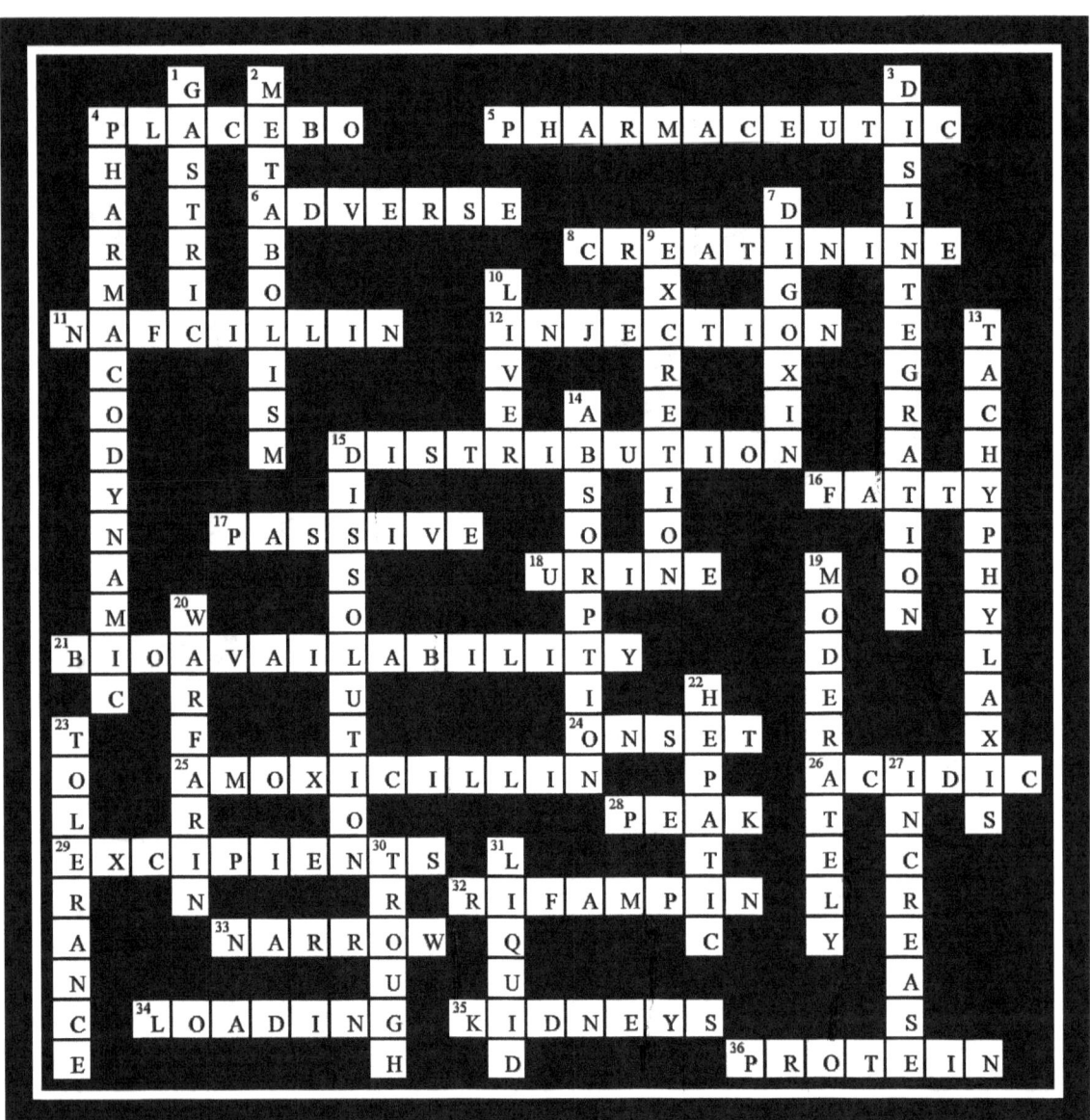

Pharmacology
Crossword Challenge
Perspectives
Drug Action
Section I
Notes

Across

4. This is given as a result of analysis of assessment data. It aids in the development of a care plan.

5. Goal setting or expected outcomes are a component of the ___ phase of the nursing process.

6. One of the factors for noncompliance may be due to a patient's ___ .

9. Some patients may respond better to this type of instruction rather than receiving printed materials.

11. The most essential component of your teaching plan is establishing a relationship of _.

12. This type of participation by the patient enhances learning.

16. An understanding of patients physiological, physical and social needs is a component of care using the ___ approach.

17. The most commonly used abbreviation for "activities of daily living."

18. This is of utmost importance because discontinuing a drug before the course is completed may result in relapse.

20. This phase of the nursing process encompasses nursing actions, and possible interventions required to achieve an outcome.

24. Information given to the patient should be tailored to their level of _.

25. Requesting the patient prepare a drug information sheet that correctly identifies their medication schedule within 5 days is an example of setting a ___ .

26. One of the top ten tips for successful teaching sessions is to remain _.

27. Symptoms verbalized by the patient are considered ___ data.

28. Those patients who are considered to be most likely to have adverse reactions are considered a ___ risk.

29. This fruit is an excellent source of potassium and recommended for those on diuretics.

30. One of the first aspects to consider when beginning the teaching process is to assess the patient for ___ .

Down

1. If goals are not met, the nursing plan may need to be ___ .

2. A diagnosis may be actual or ___ .

3. Creatinine clearance should be monitored whenever a drug is categorized as ___ .

7. Laboratory tests are one of the components considered as ___ data studied during the assessment phase of the nursing process.

8. Data collection should focus on ___ and those organs likely to be affected by drug therapy.

10. Physical health assessment, laboratory data and diagnostic studies are considered ___ studies essential for future comparisons.

13. This phase of the nursing process considers the effectiveness of teaching and attainment of goals.

14. The avoidance of large amounts of green, leafy vegetables is recommended for patients taking ___ .

15. The first phase of the nursing process.

19. The most commonly used abbreviation for North American Nursing Diagnosis Association.

21. A decrease in ___ strength may interfere with a patient's ability to open medication containers.

22. Hesitancy in taking prescribed pain medications may be due to a fear of _.

23. This sense of time addresses the importance that certain cultures place on the past, present and future.

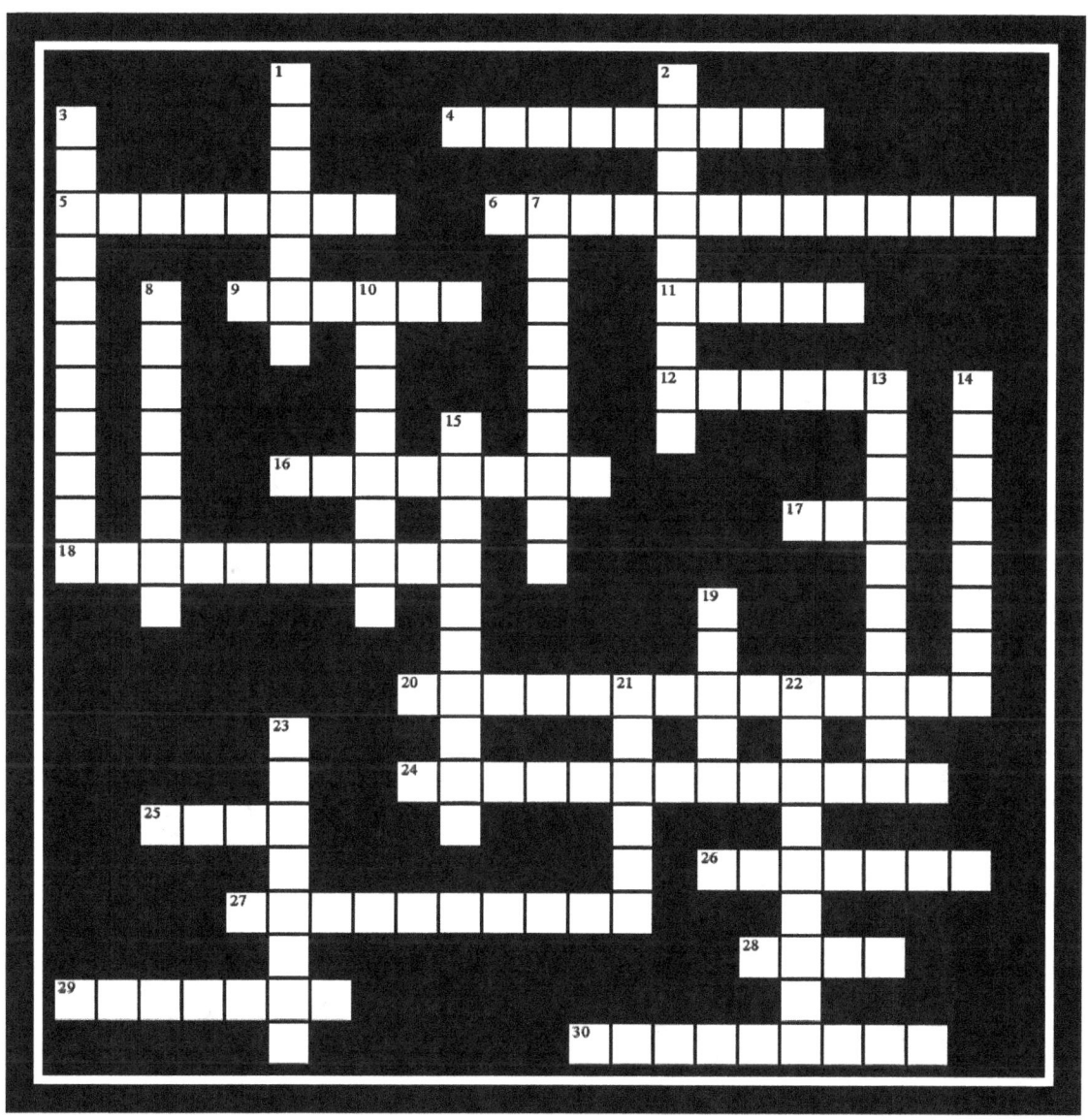

Pharmacology
Crossword Challenge
Perspectives
Nursing Process & Patient Teaching
Section I

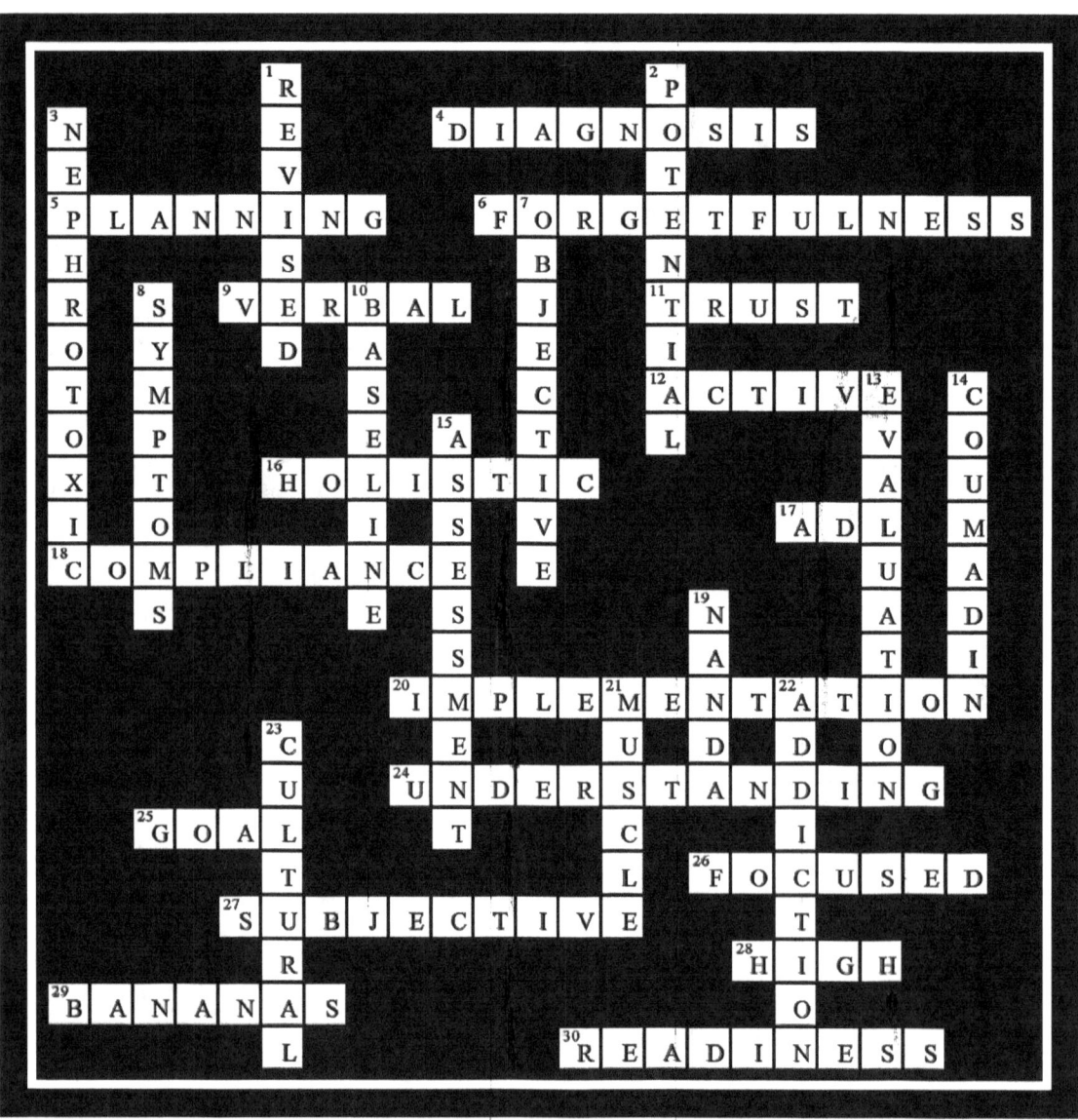

Pharmacology
Crossword Challenge
Perspectives
Nursing Process & Patient Teaching
Notes

Pharmacology
Crossword Challenge
Perspectives
Drug Administration & Principles
Section I

Across

3. According to the Joint Commission, this is not an acceptable abbreviation for ordering or documenting medications.

5. The act of drawing in the breath; drawing a medicated vapor in with the breath; a solution of a drug or combination of drugs for administration as a nebulized mist intended to reach the respiratory tree.

7. This term is used to describe a corner of the eye.

9. This category of drug orders may be an ongoing order, given for a specific number of doses or days or may have special instructions to base administration on laboratory values.

11. Do not use this site for IM injection in children.

13. An advantage of the unit dose method of drug distribution is increased ___.

15. These agents are examples of drugs that do not cross the blood-brain barrier.

16. A commonly used abbreviation for drops.

19. The typical sites for IM injections include dorsogluteal, deltoid, vastus lateralis and ___.

21. To avoid drug error, the drug label should be read ___ times.

23. The taking in, incorporation, or reception of gases, liquids, light or heat.

24. Pull down and back on the auricle when administering ear drops to ___.

26. The pattern of occurrence of a substance within or between cells, tissues, organisms.

27. A technique to estimate the amount of medication remaining in a canister is to place the canister in ___.

28. The preferred site for a medication ordered via the IM route for a 9-month old child is the vastus ___.

Down

1. The "Five-Plus-Five Rights" include the right: Client, drug, dose, assessment and ___.

2. This term describes a blister or a bleb.

4. HCT is an example of an abbreviation that is ___.

6. Needles should ___ be recapped.

8. The main route of drug excretion is via the ___.

9. This route of administration involves placing the drug under the tongue for venous absorption.

10. This effect occurs when the drug is metabolized or excreted more slowly than the rate at which it is being administered.

12. These are devices used to enhance the delivery of medications from metered-dose inhalers.

14. This is the name of the route used when placing the drug between the gum and the cheek.

17. Because IM administration is painful and may cause tissue irritation, this broad-spectrum antibiotic is typically administered orally or IV.

18. This is at the line of the desired dose.

20. A type of medication administration whereby the drug is stored in a patch which may be placed directly onto the skin.

21. This term refers to the first adverse symptoms that occur at a particular dose.

22. A box or container.

25. This method of drug distribution includes drugs that are packaged in dose for 24 hours by the pharmacy.

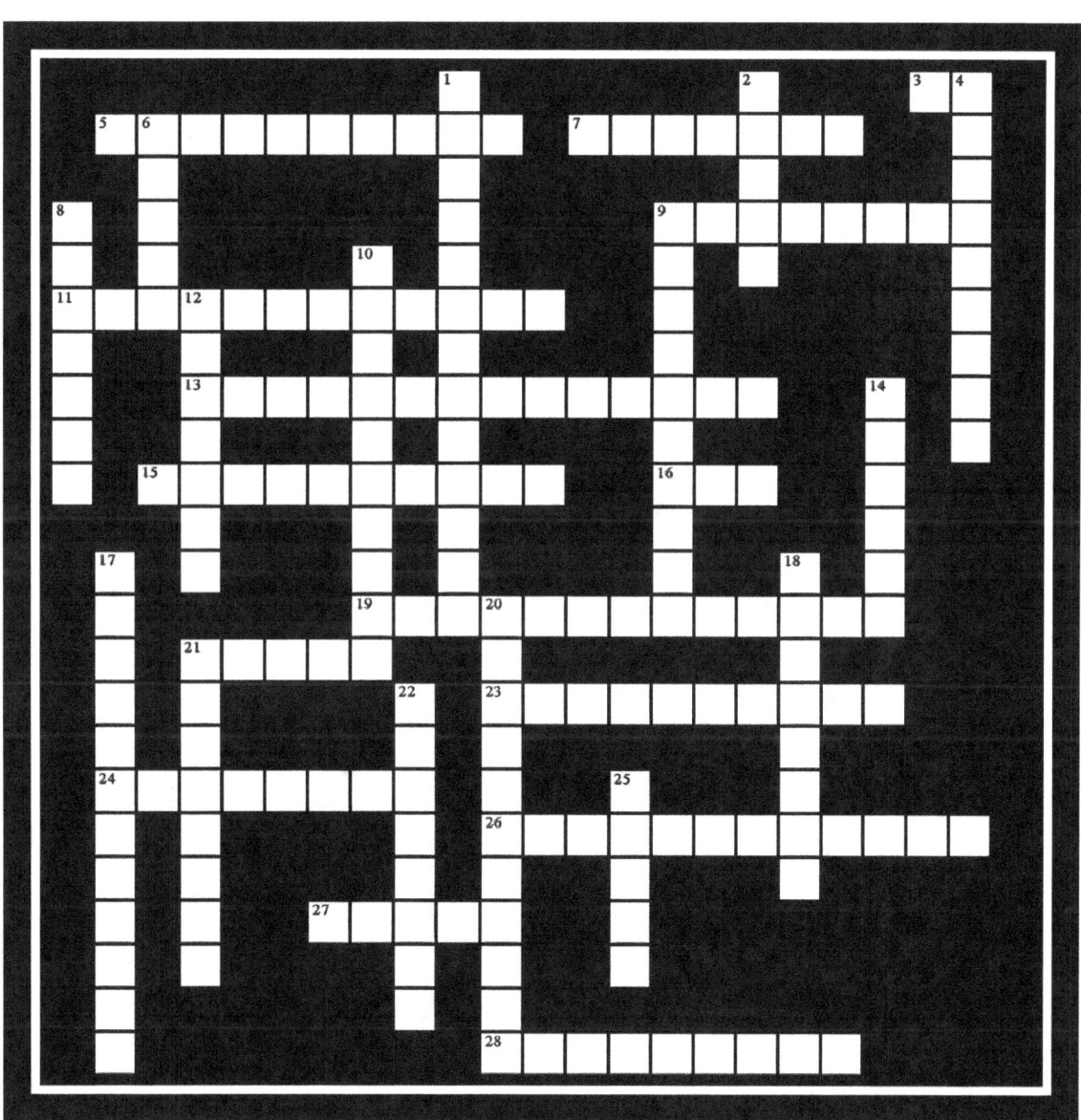

Pharmacology
Crossword Challenge
Perspectives
Drug Administration & Principles
Section I

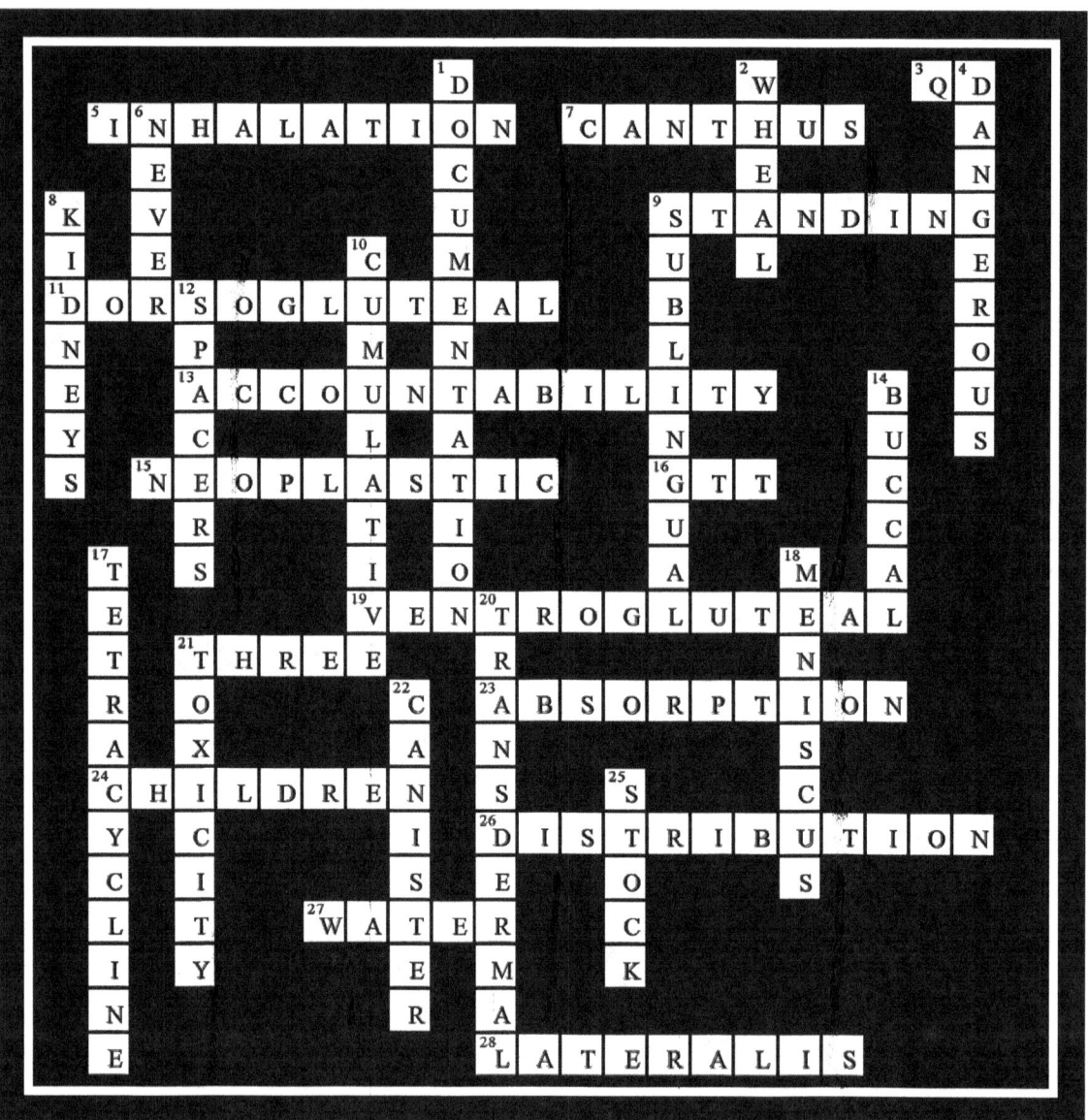

Pharmacology
Crossword Challenge
Perspectives
Drug Administration & Principles
Section I
Notes

Pharmacology
Crossword Challenge
Medication & Calculations
Section II

Across

1. A small glass container with a self-sealing rubber top.
3. ___analysis. A calculation method known as units and conversions, decreases a number of steps required to calculate a drug dosage.
5. Before calculating drug doses, all units of measure must be converted to a ___system.
7. This syringe has the capacity of 1 mL and measures in units.
8. Electronic intravenous regulators.
10. ___equation. A method similar to ratio and proportion except it is written as a fraction.
11. Commonly used abbreviation for IV piggyback.
16. This type of measurement is not as accurate as the metric system because of the lack of standardization.
19. A method of injection usually used for skin testing; diagnose the cause of an allergy.
21. A glass container with a tapered neck for snapping open and used only once.
22. IV push.
23. This syringe is a 1-mL syringe with markings in tenths and hundredths.
27. The method of injection used for a more rapid absorption.
28. This dose form is typically scored allowing it to be easily broken when half of the drug amount is needed.
29. The ounce and ___ are more frequently used for measurement of fluid volume than for dry weights.
30. This pump is programmed to administer prescribed medication at patient demand, and continuously.
31. In the apothecary system, the unit of weight is the ___.
32. This is the abbreviation for the method considered the most accurate way to calculate the drug dose for infants, children and older adults.

Down

2. This system of measurement is no longer included on any drug labels.
4. Insulin is administered this way because the absorption rate is slower.
5. ___release capsules should not be crushed /diluted because the medication will be absorbed at a much faster rate.
6. ___factor. The number of drops per mL.
9. This method is used to inject drugs into the fatty tissue for slower absorption.
12. This type of insulin is cloudy because of the substance protamine.
13. Keep vein open.
14. This may be necessary when attempting to administer an injection to a very young child.
15. The basic unit of linear measurement in the metric system.
17. This dose form is typically a gelatin shell that contains a powder or pellet.
18. This term describes medications administered intradermally, subq, IM and IV.
20. ___coated, hard-shell tablets must not be crushed because the medication may irritate the gastric mucosa.
24. The basic unit of measure for volume in the metric system.
25. The formula most frequently used when calculating drug dosages.
26. All pharmaceuticals are manufactured using this system.
31. In the metric system, this is the basic unit of measure for weight.
32. This is the abbreviation for the method of calculation which allows for the individualization of the drug dose and involves three steps.

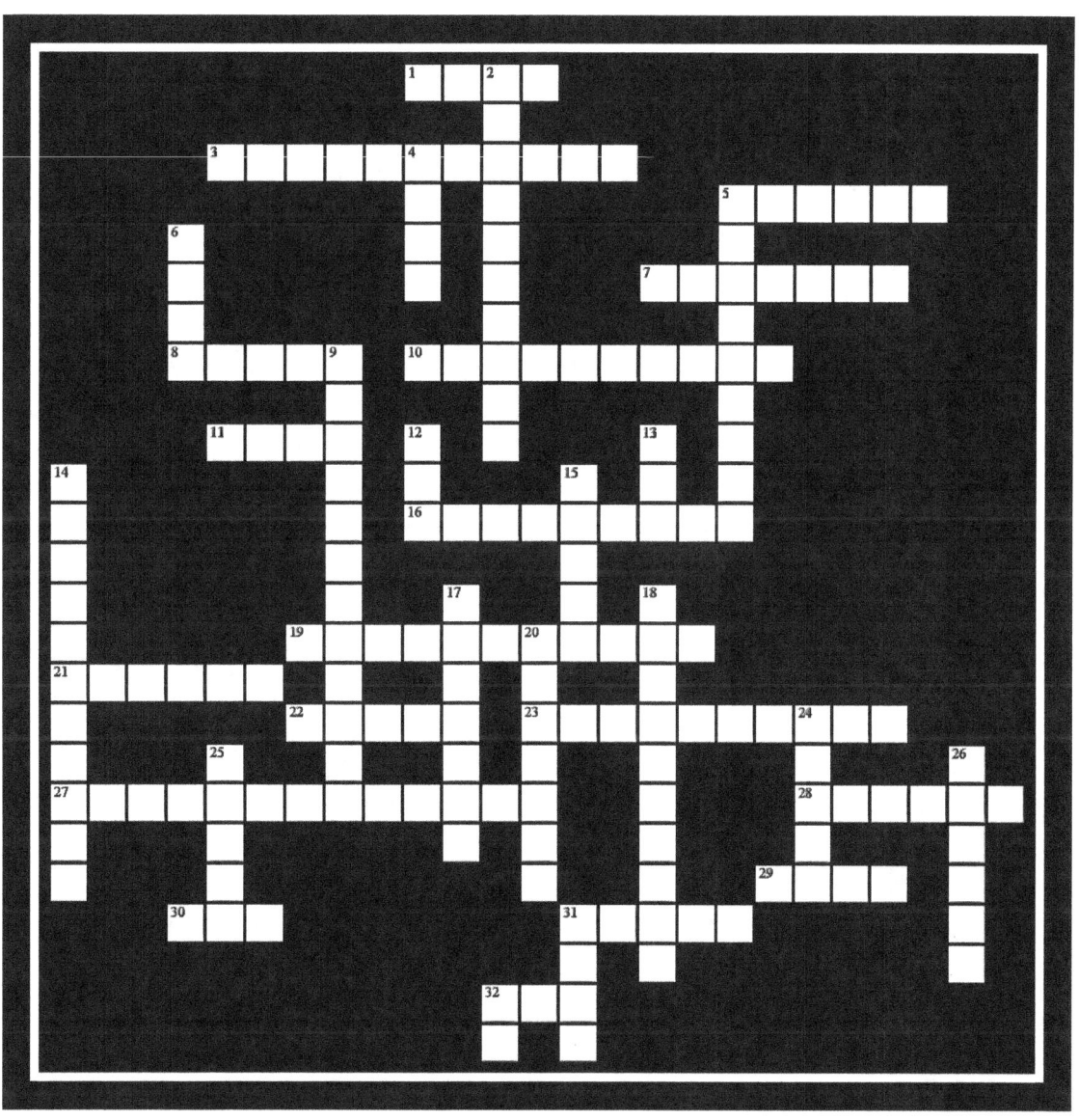

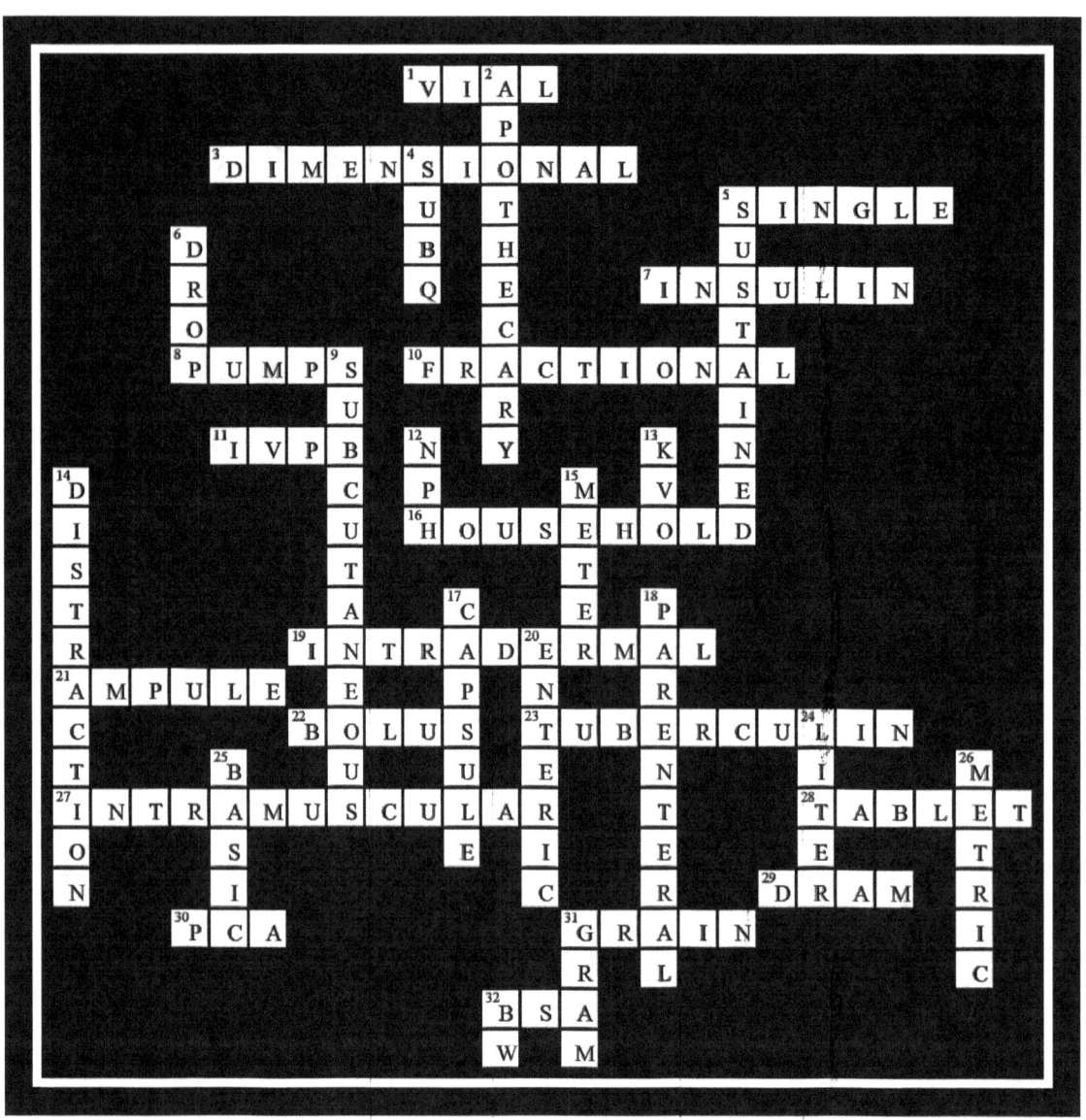

Pharmacology
Crossword Challenge
Medication & Calculations
Section II
Notes

Pharmacology
Crossword Challenge
Pharmacology Issues
Section III

Across

4. ___ecology includes concepts related to biologic variations, heredity, genetics, endemics and drug metabolism.
6. When two drugs that have opposite effects are administered together, each drug cancels the effect of the other.
11. This occurs when an additional CNS depressant is taken with alcohol, increasing the effect.
13. Serum potassium level greater than 5.3 meq/L.
18. Ferrous sulfate, gluconate or fumarate.
19. Animal studies done on category C drugs indicate a risk to ___.
20. Medicine derived from plants.
22. Vitamins A, D, E and K are considered ___ soluble.
25. The study of the time course of drug absorption, distribution, metabolism and excretion.
26. Total parenteral nutrition.
29. Synergistic drug effects act like an ___.
30. B-complex vitamins and vitamin C are ___soluble vitamins.
32. Negligence; giving the wrong drug or drug dose that results in the patient's death.
34. Drug excretion in infants and children is usually _.
35. Giving the correct drug but by the wrong route that results in the patient's death.
36. Drugs that may cause an elevated serum sodium level include ___ preparations.
37. The perspective of time, determines whether the patient stresses a past, present or future orientation.
39. This name describes the structure of chemistry: ___ structure.

Down

1. Trade name, also known as the proprietary name, registered trademark.
2. A pharmacologically inert substance.
3. The governing body empowered to monitor and regulate the manufacture and marketing of drugs.
5. Drugs that are attainable without a prescription.
7. ___distancing. Defined as the physical proximity between people conversing, varies between and among cultures.
8. Omission; omitting a drug dose that results in the patient's death.
9. ___Amendment. Legislation that increased controls on drug safety requiring adverse reactions be included on the label. (2 words)
10. A combination of ethnic and cultural variables, perceptions.
12. Negative charge.
13. Decreased serum chloride level.
14. ___psychosis. A form of amnesia characterized by loss of short-term memory and inability to learn.
15. State of being poisoned by a drug or other toxic substance.
16. Cue-induced craving may occur after long periods of ___.
17. The official, nonproprietary name for the drug.
18. This type of consent includes the participant's right to be informed and that participation is voluntary.
21. Brain reward system.
23. When a patient takes a hepatic-enzyme inducer, the dose of the warfarin is usually ___.
24. Fluid which has more particles than water.
25. Administration of many drugs together.
27. When two drugs with similar action are administered, the drug interaction is called an ___ effect.
28. This type of drug reaction is an undesirable drug effect that ranges from mild-to-severe effects.
29. A drug information reference that provides accurate & complete drug data on nearly all US prescription drugs.
31. Serotonin antagonist (herb) that relieves migraine headaches.
33. Vitamin D has a major role in regulating ___.
38. According to US standards, the highest potential for drug abuse is found in this schedule.

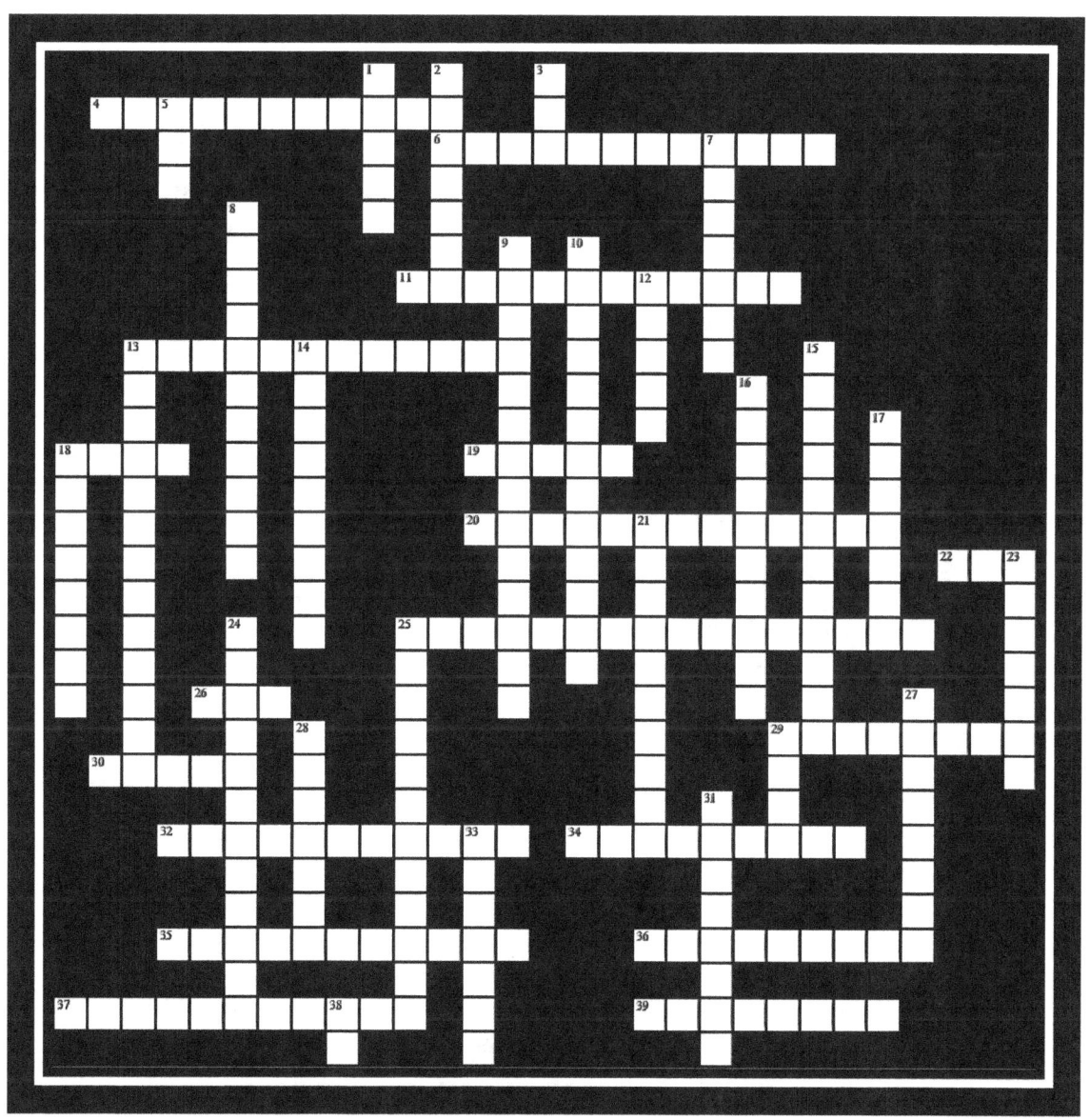

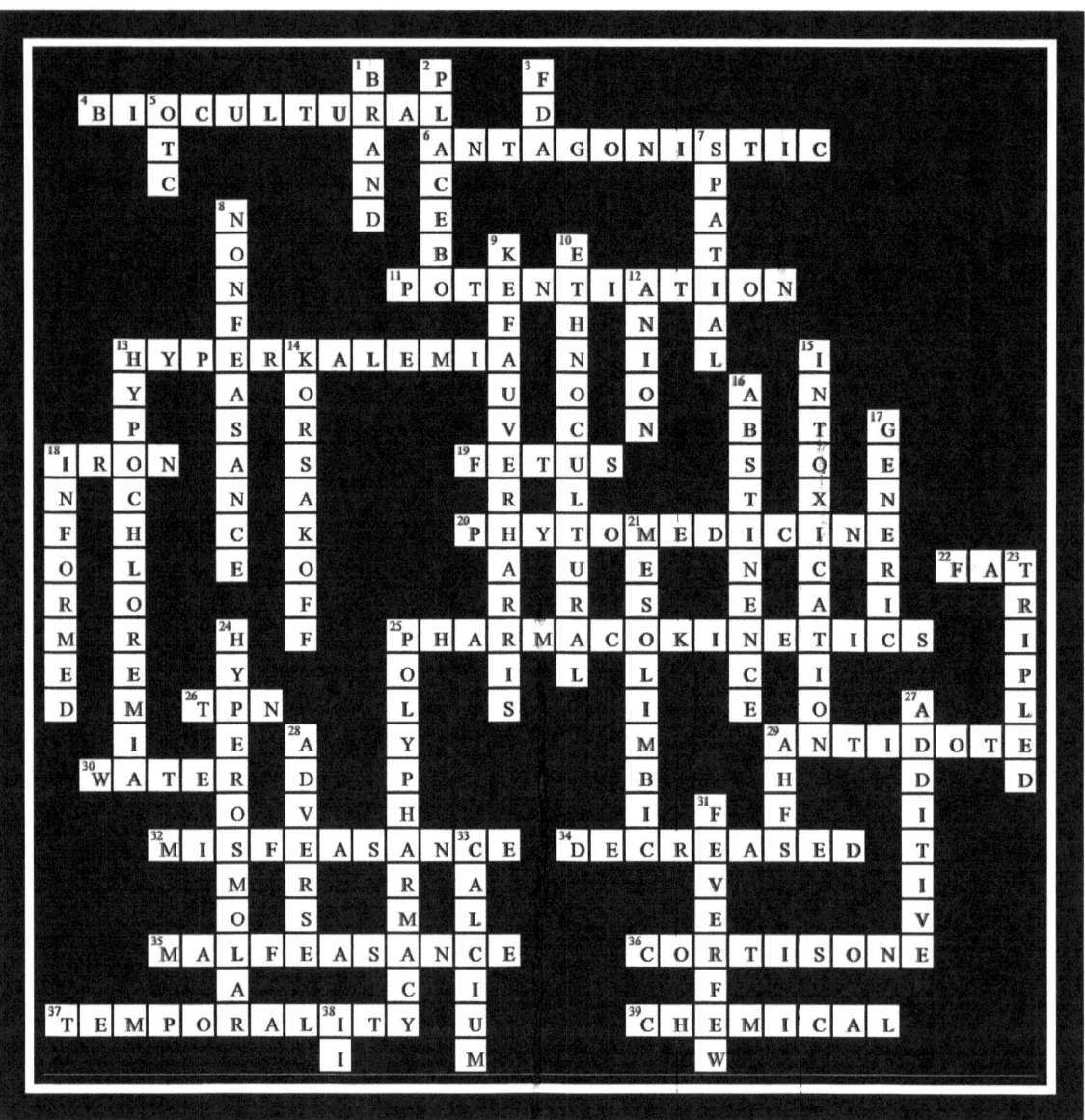

Pharmacology
Crossword Challenge
Pharmacology Issues
Section III
Notes

Across

4. Benztropine is a drug used to treat ___ disease.
6. Bethanechol is a drug used to treat ___ retention.
7. Central nervous system.
8. Patients taking albuterol should be monitored for ___.
11. A sympathetic response on the bladder will cause it to ___.
12. A parasympathetic effect on the eye will cause it to ___.
13. This neurotransmitter at the end of a neuron innervates muscle.
15. This drug may cause a drug interaction in patients taking epinephrine.
19. This catecholamine hormone is released from the terminal nerve ending and stimulates the cell receptors to produce a response.
20. This system is also called the sympathetic nervous system.
21. Efferent neurons are also referred to as ___ neurons.
22. Alpha blockers promote vasodilation and a ___ in blood pressure.
23. Adrenergic blockers.
24. Dilation of the pupils.
25. Chemical structures of a substance that can produce a sympathomimetic response.

Down

1. This receptor stimulates smooth muscle and slows the heart rate.
2. Constriction of the pupils.
3. Drugs that block the effects of the adrenergic neurotransmitter are called adrenergic ___.
4. This drug is a direct-acting cholinergic that constricts the pupils. It is used to treat glaucoma.
5. Isopropamide is a drug used to treat ___ .
9. Peripheral nervous system.
10. Drugs that inhibit the actions of acetylcholine by occupying the acetylcholine receptors are called ___.
13. Autonomic nervous system.
14. Indirect-acting cholinergic drugs inhibit the action of this enzyme.
16. Sensory neurons are also referred to as ___ neurons.
17. Patients should be monitored for ___ when taking metoprolol.
18. The central nervous system includes the spinal cord and the ___.
19. This receptor affects skeletal muscles.

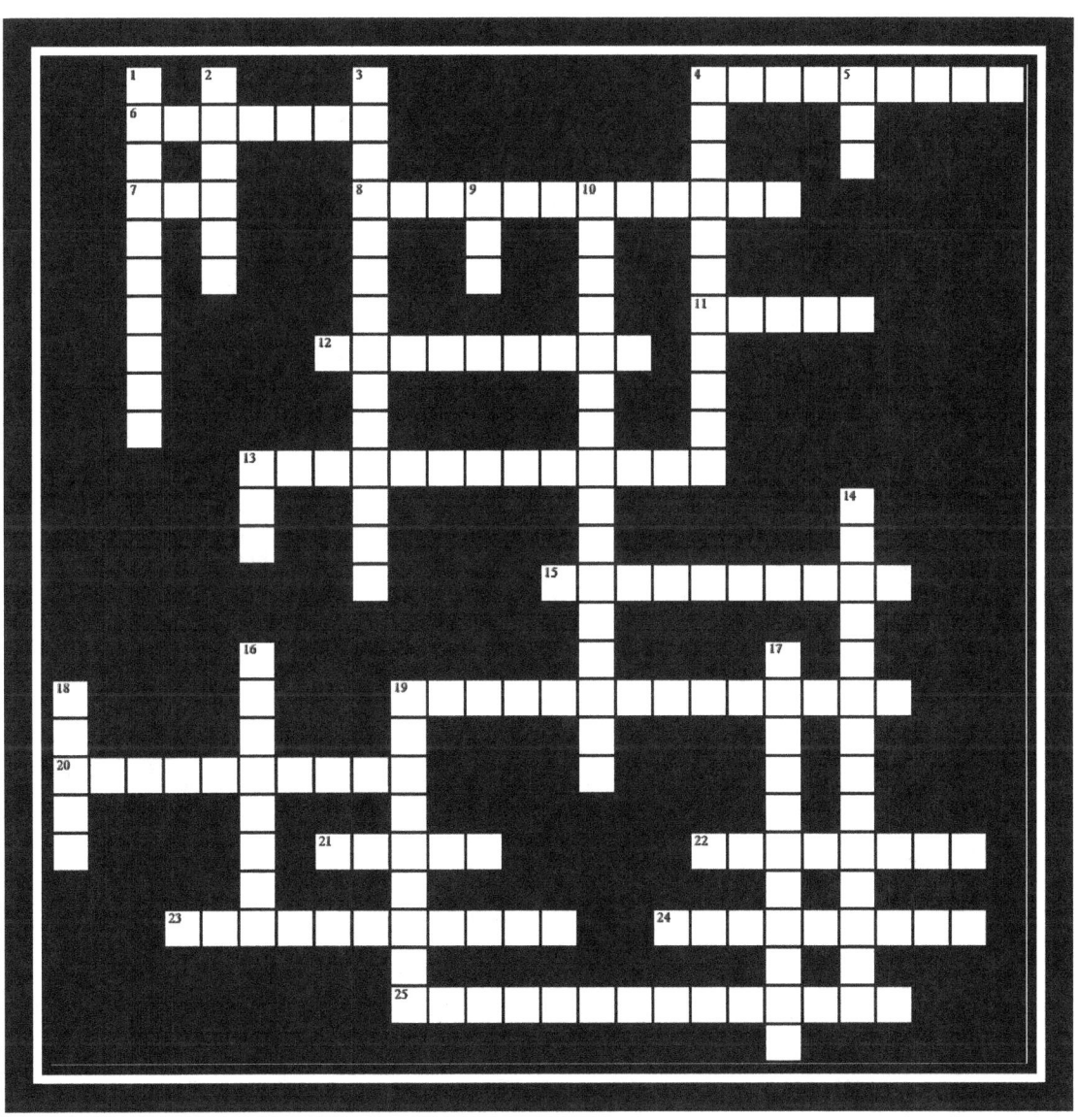

Pharmacology
Crossword Challenge
Autonomic Nervous System
Autonomic Nervous System Agents
Section IV

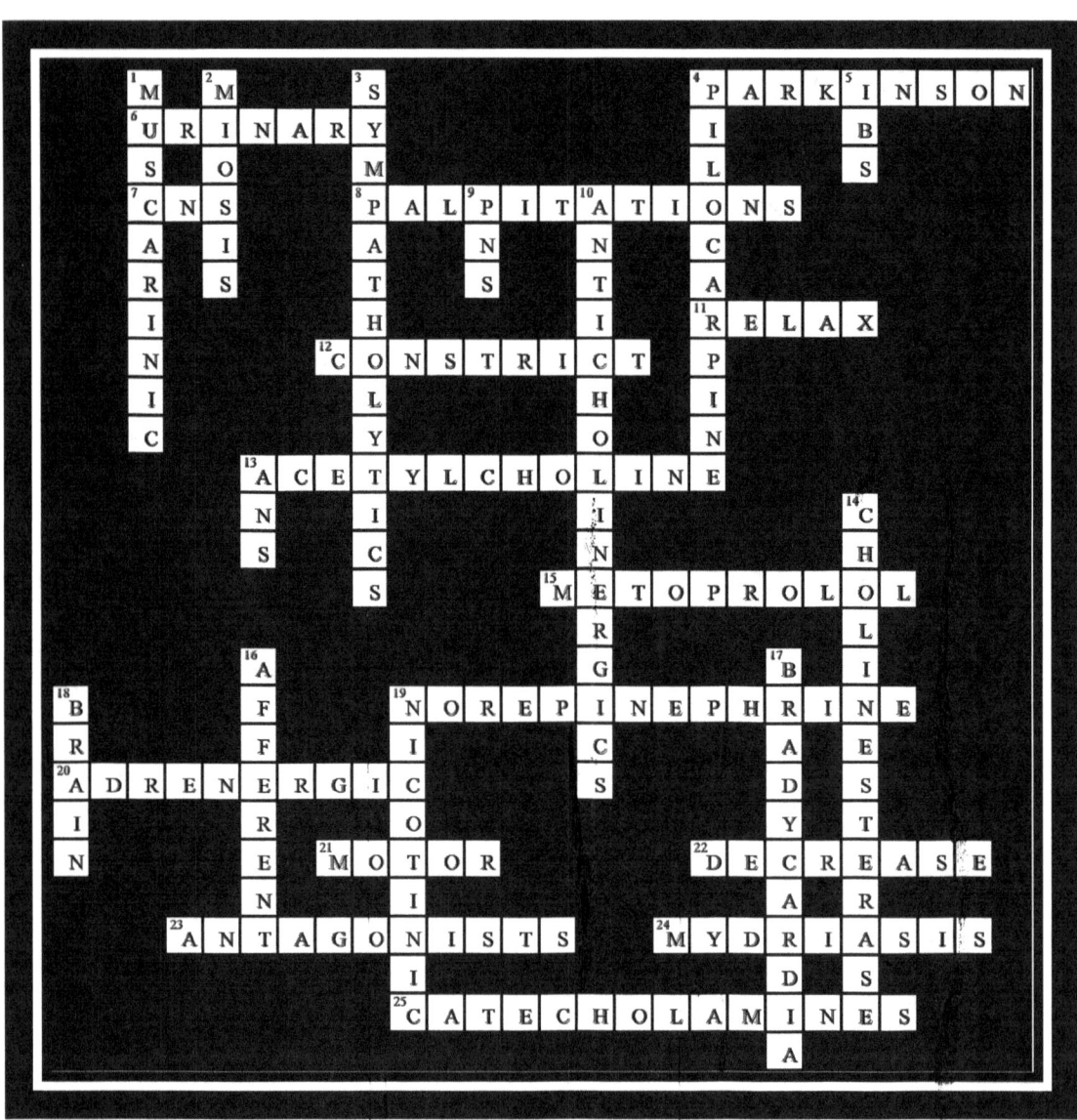

Pharmacology
Crossword Challenge
Autonomic Nervous System
Autonomic Nervous System Agents
Section IV
Notes

Across

1. Hyoscyamine. Treatment of peptic ulcer and IBS. Controls gastric secretion and spastic bladder.
4. An example of a mixed-acting sympathomimetic which acts indirectly by stimulating the release of norepinephrine from the nerve terminals.
9. Terbutaline. Bronchodilator. Used to correct bronchospasms.
10. Monoamine oxidase, inside the neuron, one of two enzymes that inactivates the metabolism of norepinephrine.
11. Ipratropium bromide. Bronchodilator used to treat COPD.
12. Coreg (carvedilol) is an example of an ___ blocker.
14. Inderal. Used for management of angina pectoris, MI, HBP, dysrhythmias.
15. The principal use of this drug is to promote micturition.
16. Corgard. Used in management of hypertension and angina pectoris.
19. Treats cardiac decompensation by enhancing myocardial contractility, stroke volume and cardiac output.
21. Cognex. Used to improve memory in mild-to-moderate Alzherimer's dementia.
24. Betapace. Used to treat life-threatening ventricular arrhythmias and chronic angina pectoris.
25. The primary reaction of albuterol is on the ___ receptor.
26. ProAmatine. A drug used to treat symptomatic orthostatic hypotension.

Down

2. Cholinergics ___ the parasympathetic nervous system.
3. One of the effects of cholinergic drugs on the cardiovascular system is that it ___ heart rate.
5. Prostigmin. Used to increase muscle strength in myasthenia gravis.
6. A preoperative medication used to reduce salivation, increase heart rate and dilate pupils. It inhibits acetylcholine.
7. Trade name for albuterol.
8. This drug is frequently used in emergencies to treat anaphylaxis. It is a potent inotropic that increases cardiac output.
12. This drug produces a bronchodilation effect.
13. Used primarily to treat hypertension, it regulates the release of norepinephrine by inhibiting its release.
14. Minipress. Used for management of mild-to-moderate hypertension.
17. Norepinephrine. Used for shock, is a potent vasoconstrictor.
18. Abbreviation for Catechol-O-methyltransferase, outside the neuron. One of two enzymes that inactivate the metabolism of norepinephrine.
20. Used for treatment of SVT, atrial fibrillation and HTN.
22. Trihexyphenidyl. Used to decrease involuntary symptoms of parkinsonism.
23. Beta receptors are located primarily in the ___ .

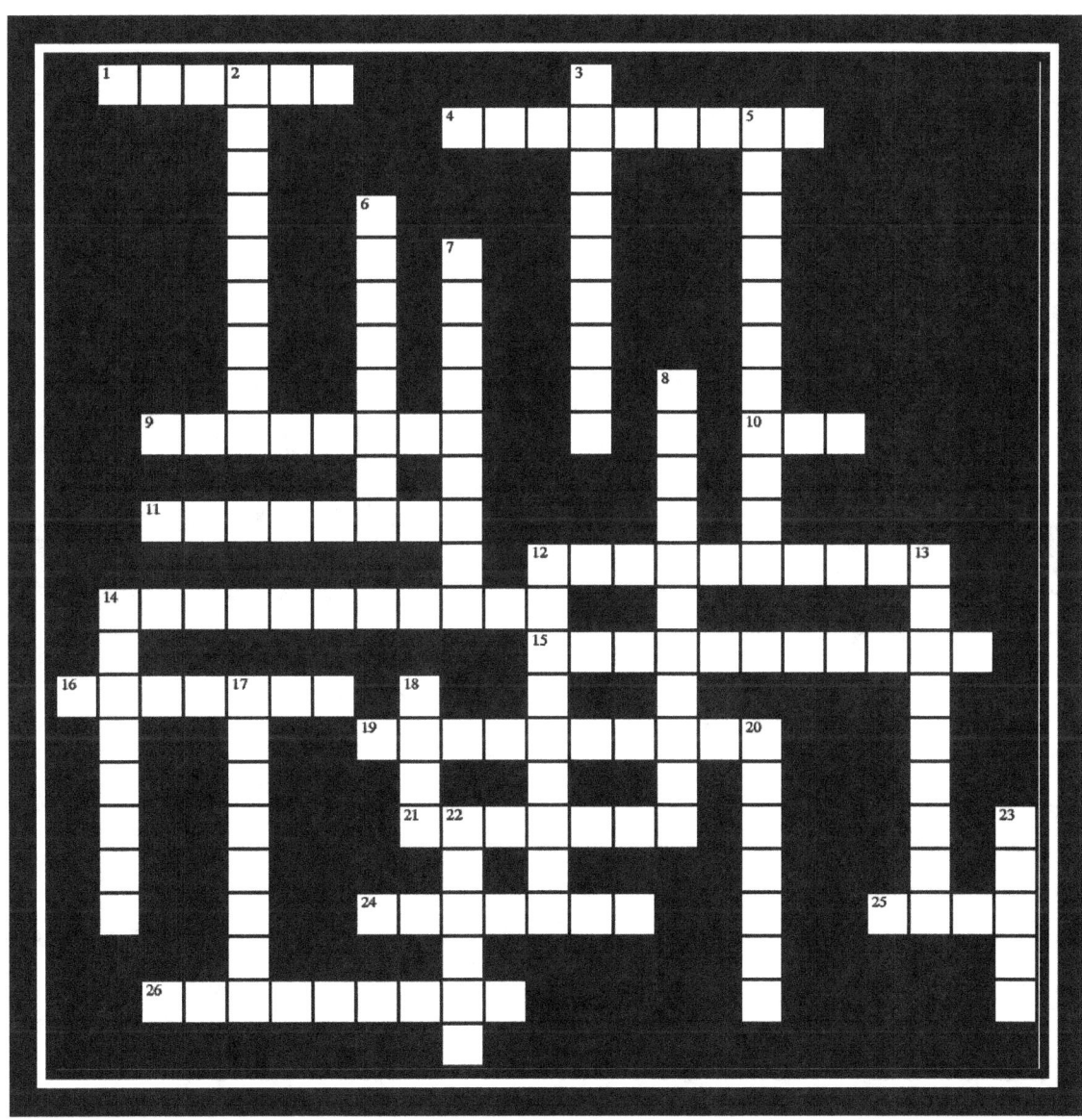

Pharmacology
Crossword Challenge
Autonomic Nervous System
Drugs and Drug Action
Section IV

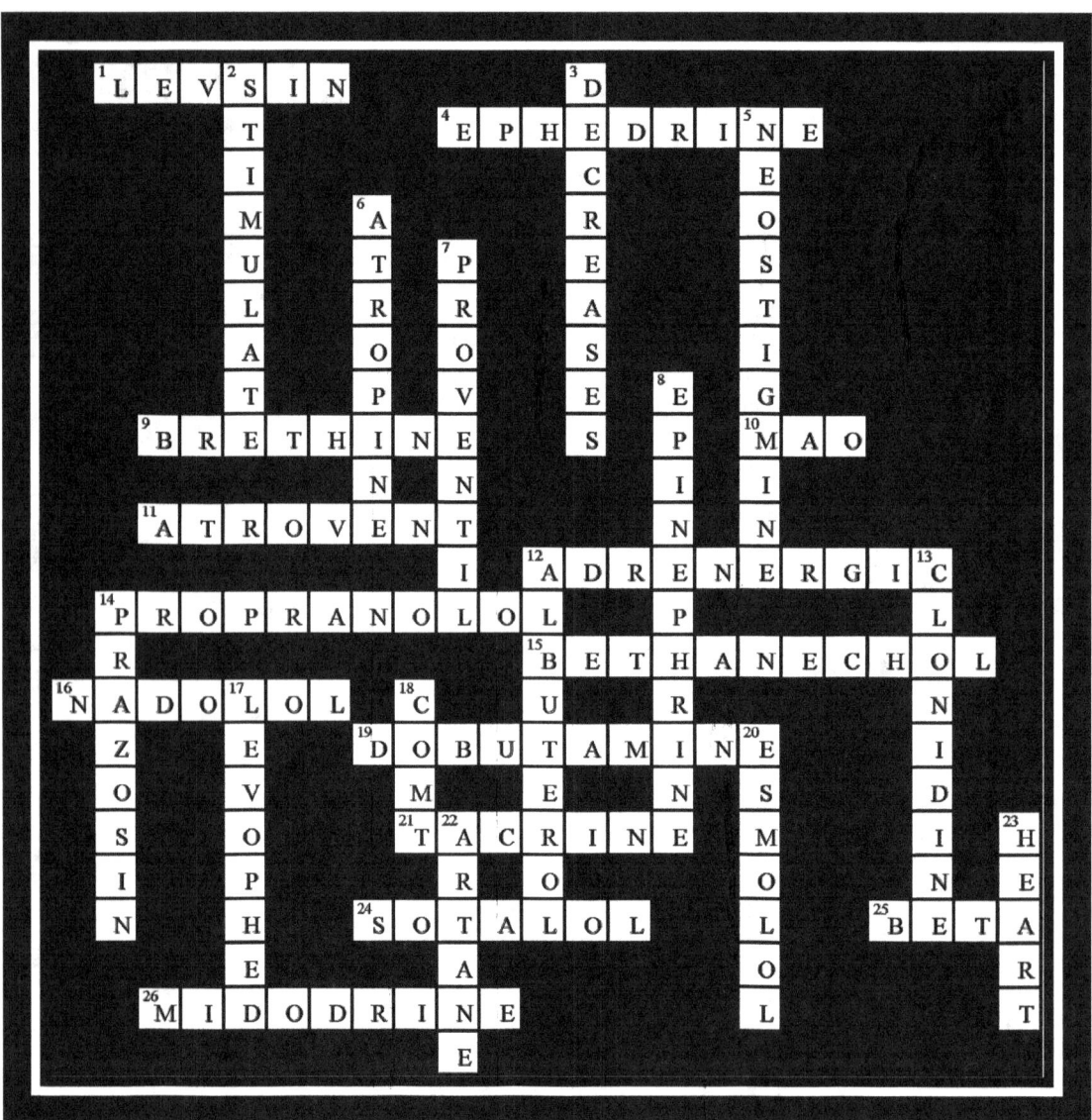

Pharmacology
Crossword Challenge
Autonomic Nervous System
Drugs and Drug Action
Section IV
Notes

Pharmacology
Crossword Challenge
Neurologic & Neuromuscular Agents
CNS Stimulants
Section V

Across

3. A common side effect of analeptics.
7. These stimulate the release of neurotransmitters from the brain and sympathetic nervous system.
8. Generic name for Imitrex. Adverse reaction, life-threatening, may cause coronary artery vasospasm, MI, cardiac arrest.
11. This condition is characterized by falling asleep during normal waking activities such as driving a car or talking.
13. Generic name for Amerge. Given for acute migraines, causes vasoconstriction of cranial carotid arteries.
15. Triptans. ___agonists, (5-HT)
16. These drugs treat migraine attacks.
18. This drug is typically given to increase a child's attention span and cognitive performance.
20. Not for prolonged use, but given to prevent or abort migraine attacks.
23. Given through an NG tube, may be used for newborns with apnea to stimulate respiration.
25. Commonly used abbreviation for attention deficit/hyperactivity disorder.
26. Because organs are innervated by both the sympathetic and parasympathetic systems, they can produce ___ responses.
28. The sympathetic nervous system is also called the ___ division of the ANS.
29. The purpose of the nervous system is to receive stimuli and ___ information.

Down

1. This headache is characterized by a severe unilateral nonthrobbing pain usually located around the eye.
2. Methylphenidate is well absorbed from the ___ mucosa.
4. Excessive motility, or muscular activity.
5. The nervous system is composed of all nerve tissues: brain, spinal cord, nerves, and ___.
6. An analeptic used for newborns with apnea to stimulate respiration.
9. Used to treat respiratory depression caused by drug overdose.
10. A condition in which larger and larger doses of a drug are needed to reproduce the initial response.
12. The PNS consists of two divisions: the autonomic nervous system and the ___ nervous system.
14. The primary use of an analeptic is to stimulate ___.
17. The term used to describe appetite suppressants.
19. These CNS stimulants mostly affect the brainstem and spinal cord but also affect the cerebral cortex.
21. The generic name for Adipex. Given for appetite suppression.
22. The generic name for Provigil. Used in the treatment of narcolepsy.
24. The excretion of amphetamines is ___ in urine.
27. Abbreviation for protein binding.

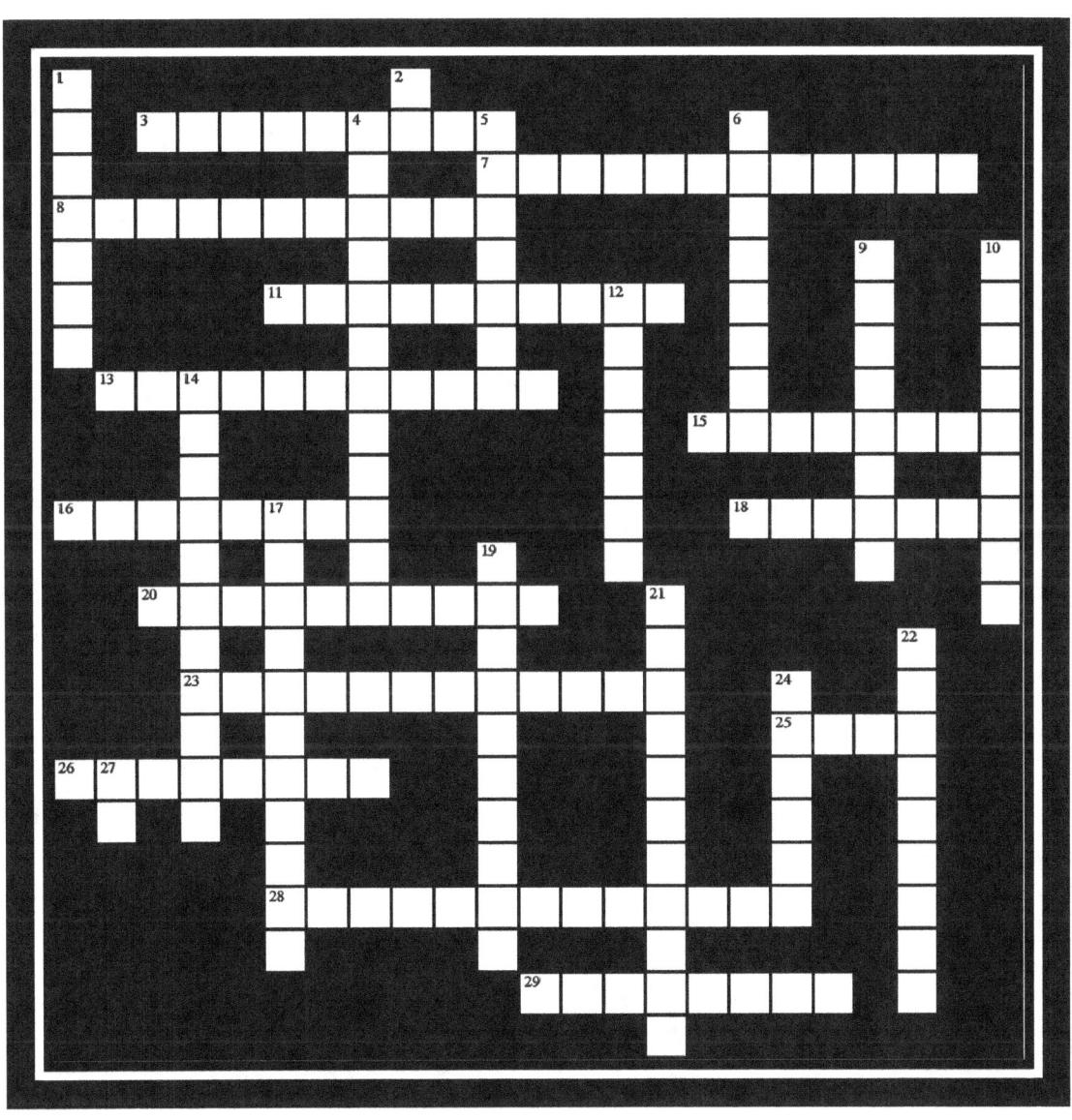

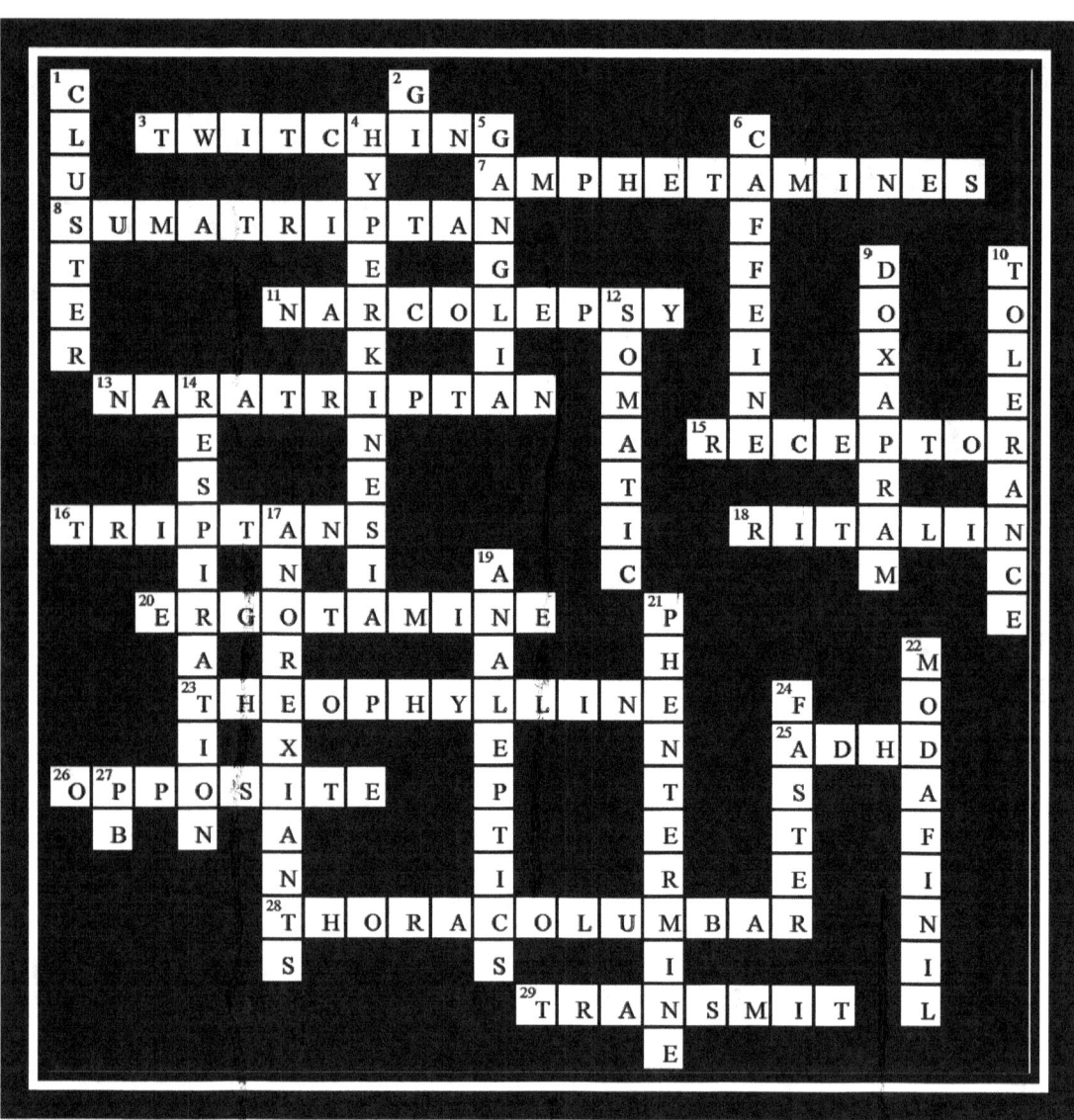

Pharmacology
Crossword Challenge
Neurologic & Neuromuscular Agents
CNS Stimulants
Section V
Notes

Across

  2. Medullary paralysis. This is the fourth and ___ stage of anesthesia.
  6. Used as a local anesthetic, this block is placed near the sacrum.
  9. The generic name for Ambien. Used for insomnia, this drug is classified as a nonbenzodiazepine.
 10. Forane. Not to be used as inhalation therapy during labor as it suppresses uterine contractions.
 11. The generic name for Butisol. Relieves anxiety and as a short-term hypnotic for insomnia.
 14. The generic name for Nembutal. Used for sedation, sleep or preanesthetic.
 16. The generic name for Lunesta. Treats insomnia.
 20. The generic name for Romazicon. used in the management of benzodiazepine overdose.
 22. The generic name for Zolpidem may lead to this type of dependence.
 24. The generic name for Xanax. Used for alleviating anxiety that may cause sleeplessness.
 25. The abbreviation for rapid eye movement.
 27. A compound that reversibly depresses neuronal function, producing loss of ability to perceive pain and/or other sensations.
 28. Diprivan. Used for induction of anesthesia. Short duration of action. May cause hypotension and respiratory depression.

Down

  1. The generic name for Versed. Used for induction of anesthesia and for endoscopic procedures.
  3. During the third stage of anesthesia, a gas or volatile liquid is administered as an ___ anesthetic.
  4. This local anesthetic block is given at the lower end of the spinal column.
  5. A derivative of barbituric acid, including phenobarbital and others, that act as CNS depressants and are used for their tranquilizing, hypnotic, and anti-seizure effects.
  7. The generic for Seconal. A short-acting drug that may cause one to awaken early in the morning.
  8. The mildest form of CNS depression, diminishes physical and mental responses.
 12. The placement of this local anesthetic is in the outer covering of the spinal cord, or the dura mater.
 13. For outpatient surgery of short duration, this type of anesthetic might be the preferred form of anesthesia.
 15. The use of these anesthetics is limited to mucous membranes, broken or unbroken skin surfaces and burns.
 17. The inability to fall asleep.
 18. Xylocaine. Introduced in 1948 as a nerve block, infiltration, epidural and spinal anesthesias.
 19. The generic name for Placidyl. Barbiturate-like drug used for sedation and sleep.
 20. General anesthesia proceeds through ___ stages.
 21. The generic name for ProSom. New benzodiazepine hypnotic for treatment of insomnia.
 23. The generic name for Ativan. A benzodiazepine that acts by increasing the action of inhibitory neurotransmitter GABA to GABA receptor.
 26. The surgical procedure is performed during this stage of anesthesia.

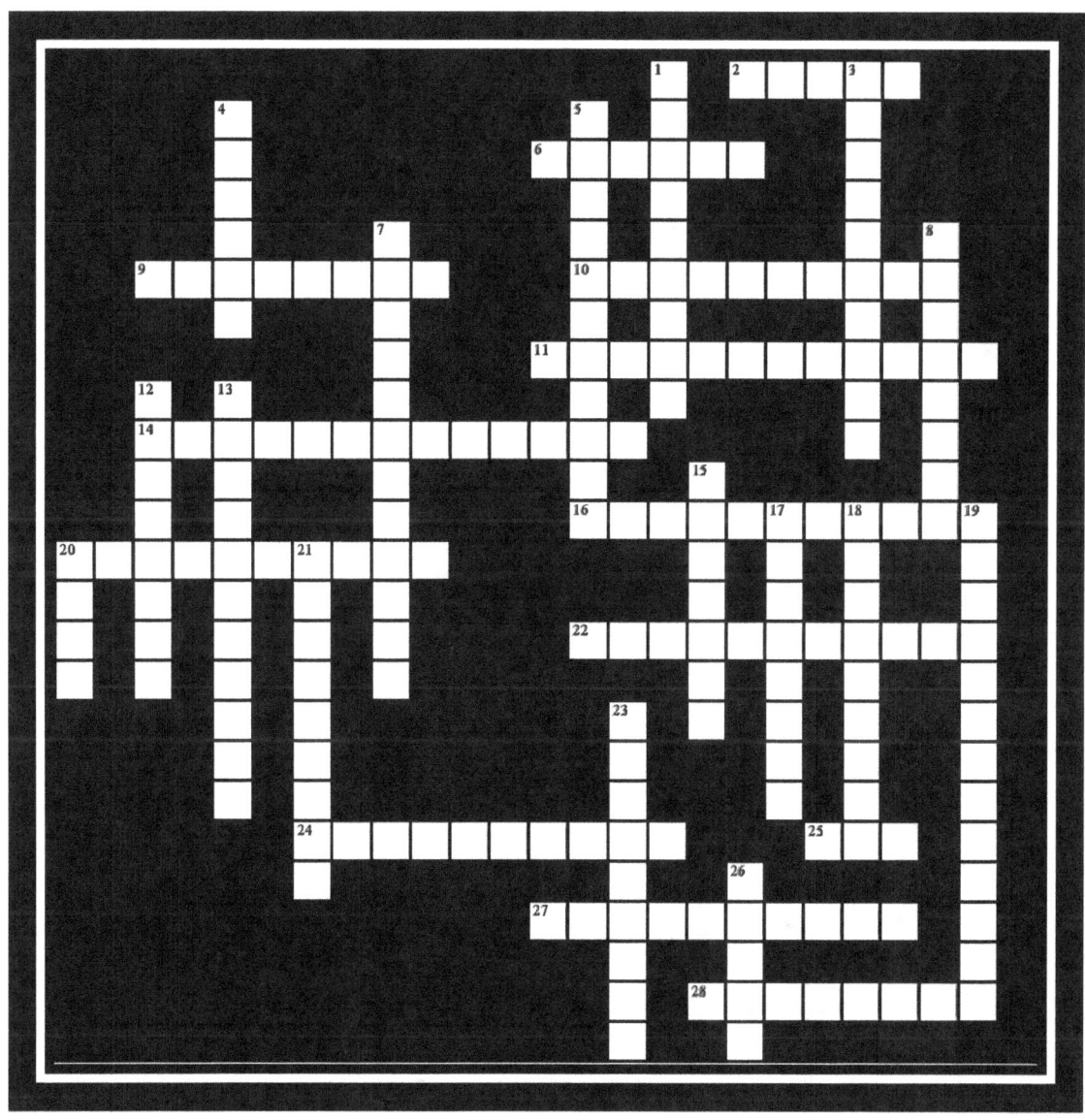

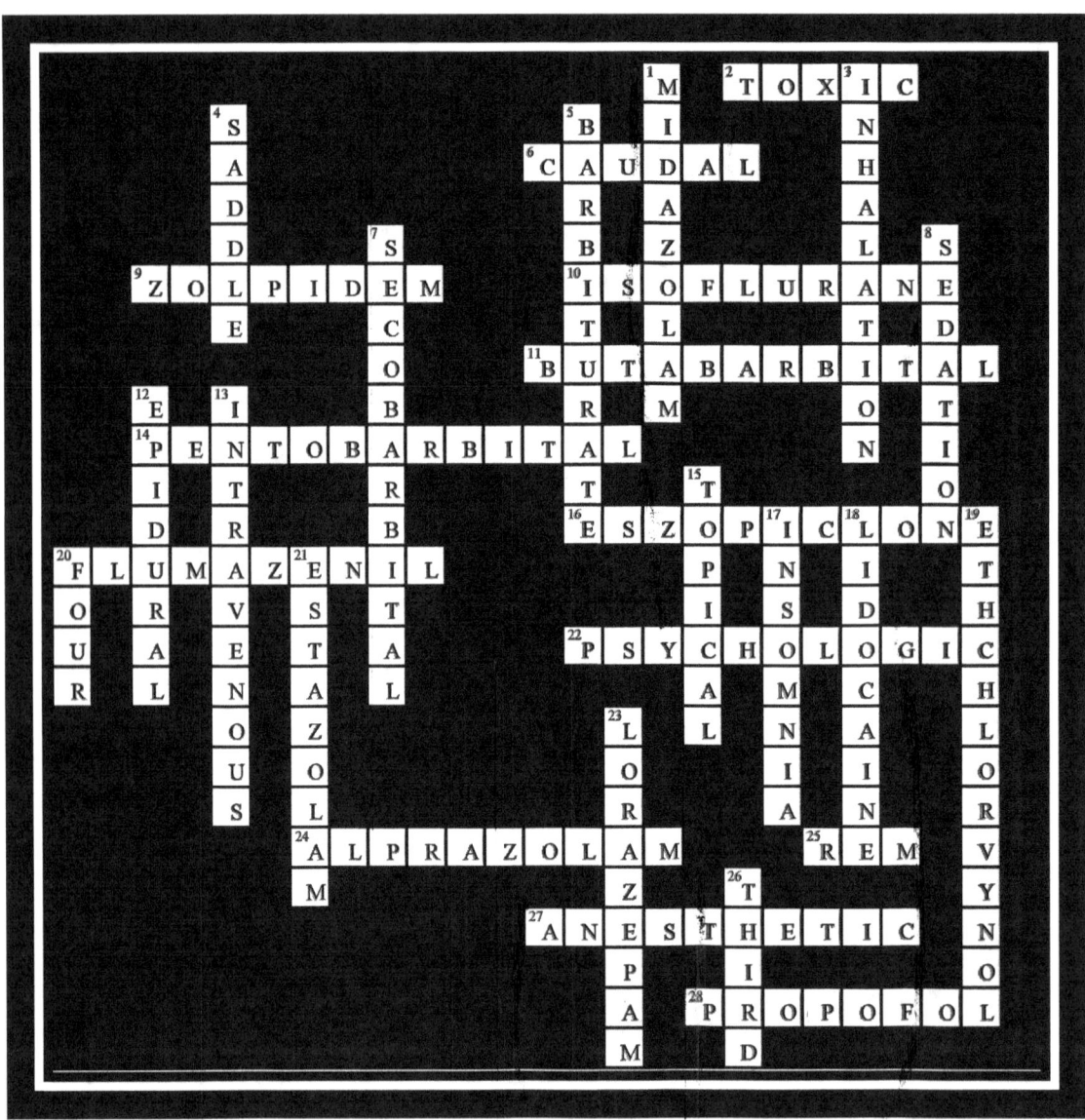

Pharmacology
Crossword Challenge
Neurologic & Neuromuscular Agents
CNS Depressants
Section V
Notes

Across

6. A brand name for trihexyphenidyl.
7. This tonic-clonic seizure is the most common form where skeletal muscles contract or tighten followed by jerkiness. ___ mal.
8. This type of seizure causes sustained muscle contractions.
9. The generic name for Azilect. Interferes with dopamine reuptake at synapses in the brain.
10. A severe side effect of hydantoins includes overgrowth of gum tissues, reddened gums that bleed easily, ___ hyperplasia.
12. These agents act by inhibiting sodium influx, stabilizing cell membranes.
14. A neurotransmitter, a depletion of which causes parkinsonism.
16. This disease is an incurable dementia illness characterized by chronic, progressive neurodegenerative conditions with marked cognitive dysfunction.
17. A trade name for carbidopa-levodopa, dopaminergic, relieves tremors and rigidity.
18. Rapid succession of epileptic seizures, status ___.
19. This enzyme inactivates dopamine.
20. Drugs used for epileptic seizures.
22. Absence seizure. It causes a brief loss of consciousness, fewer than three spike waves on the EEG, usually occurs in children, ___ mal.
23. The generic name for Norflex. Used for treatment of parkinsonism, antihistamine with anticholinergic effects.
25. Another term for "of unknown origin."
26. The abbreviation for gamma-aminobutyric acid.

Down

1. Absence of oxygen.
2. The generic term for Comtan. A COMT inhibitor, increases concentration of levodopa.
3. The generic term for Eldepryl. Inhibits the catabolic enzymes of dopamine.
4. Slow movement.
5. A chronic neurologic disorder that affects the extrapyramidal motor tract.
8. Causing abnormal prenatal development.
11. Constant, involuntary, cyclical movement of the eyeball.
13. Dopaminergics and anticholinergics are contraindicated in clients with ___.
14. Impaired voluntary movement.
15. The generic term for Dilantin.
21. This type of seizure is characterized by sustained muscle contraction.
24. A recording of the abnormal electric discharges of the cerebral cortex.

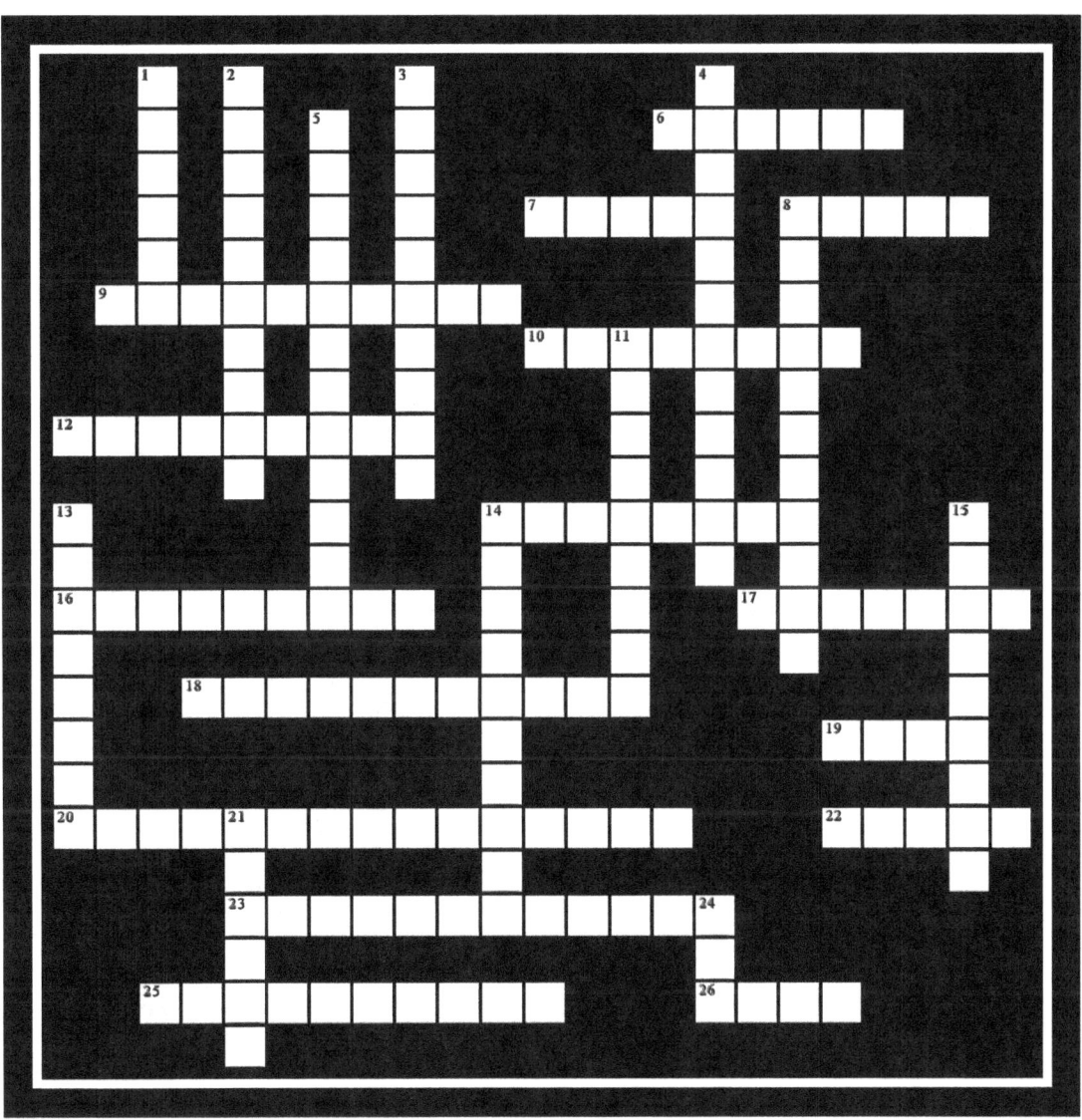

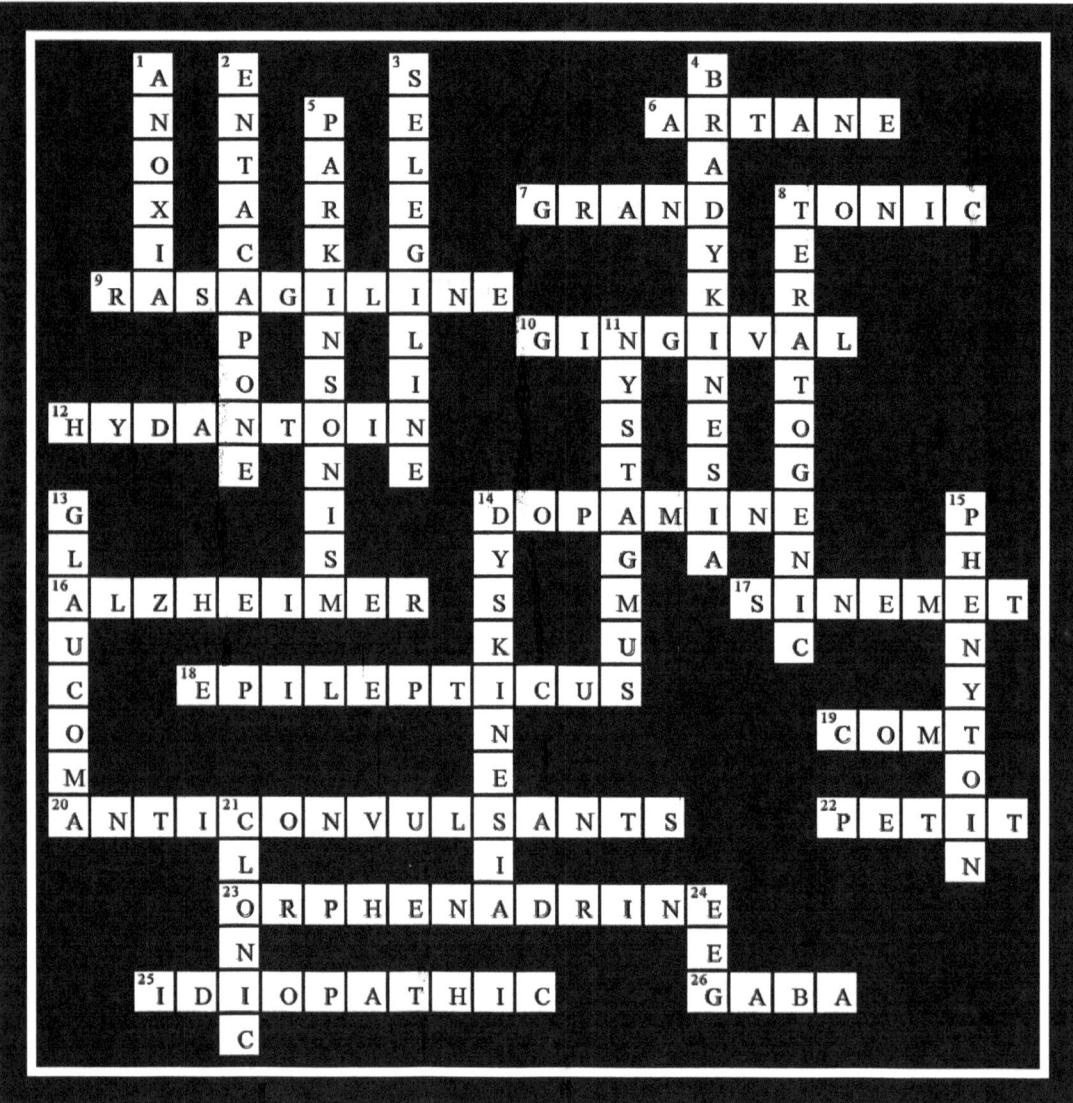

Pharmacology
Crossword Challenge
Neurologic & Neuromuscular Agents
Anticonvulsants & Neurologic Disorders
Section V
Notes

Across

1. An adverse reaction to pyridostigmine administration may cause this.
6. Kava kava and valerian herbal supplements may potentiate central nervous system depression with the administration of this drug.
7. Paralysis of both lower extremities and generally, the lower trunk.
9. Pyridostigmine is ___ absorbed from the GI tract.
12. It is important to avoid confusing baclofen, a muscle relaxant, with Beclovent which is a corticosteroid ___.
14. The generic name for Mestinon. Used in the treatment for myasthenia gravis.
15. The generic name for Prostigmin. A short-acting AChE inhibitor.
20. A brand name for cyclophosphamide. This drug is helpful for patients with multiple sclerosis in the chronic progressive phase.
21. The generic name for Skelaxin. Used in the treatment of acute, painful muscle spasticity.
22. An acute exacerbation of symptoms, ___ crisis.
23. The term used to describe abnormal pupil constriction.
24. The generic name for Imuran. May be used in conjunction with lower doses of prednisone.
25. Involuntary muscle twitching.

Down

2. Trade name for orphenadrine.
3. ___ inhibitor, (AChE). The cholinesterases that hydrolyze acetylcholine to acetate and choline within the central nervous system.
4. Muscle spasms have various causes, including injury or motor ___ disorders.
5. The term used to describe difficulty breathing.
8. A drug in this category, when administered, helps to relieve muscle spasms.
10. Spasticity of muscles can be reduced with the use of skeletal muscle ___.
11. This drug might be prescribed to treat spasticity following a spinal cord injury.
13. This phase of MS is progressive, typically characterized as wheelchair bound.
16. Another term for cerebral vascular accident.
17. A disorder of neuromuscular transmission marked by fluctuating weakness and fatigue of certain voluntary muscles. ___ gravis.
18. This is a group of drugs used to control myasthenia gravis.
19. This term describes difficulty swallowing.
21. Common demyelinating disorder of the central nervous system, causing patches of sclerosis (plaques) in the brain and spinal cord. ___ sclerosis.
22. When muscular weakness of the patient with MG becomes generalized, myasthenic ___ may occur.

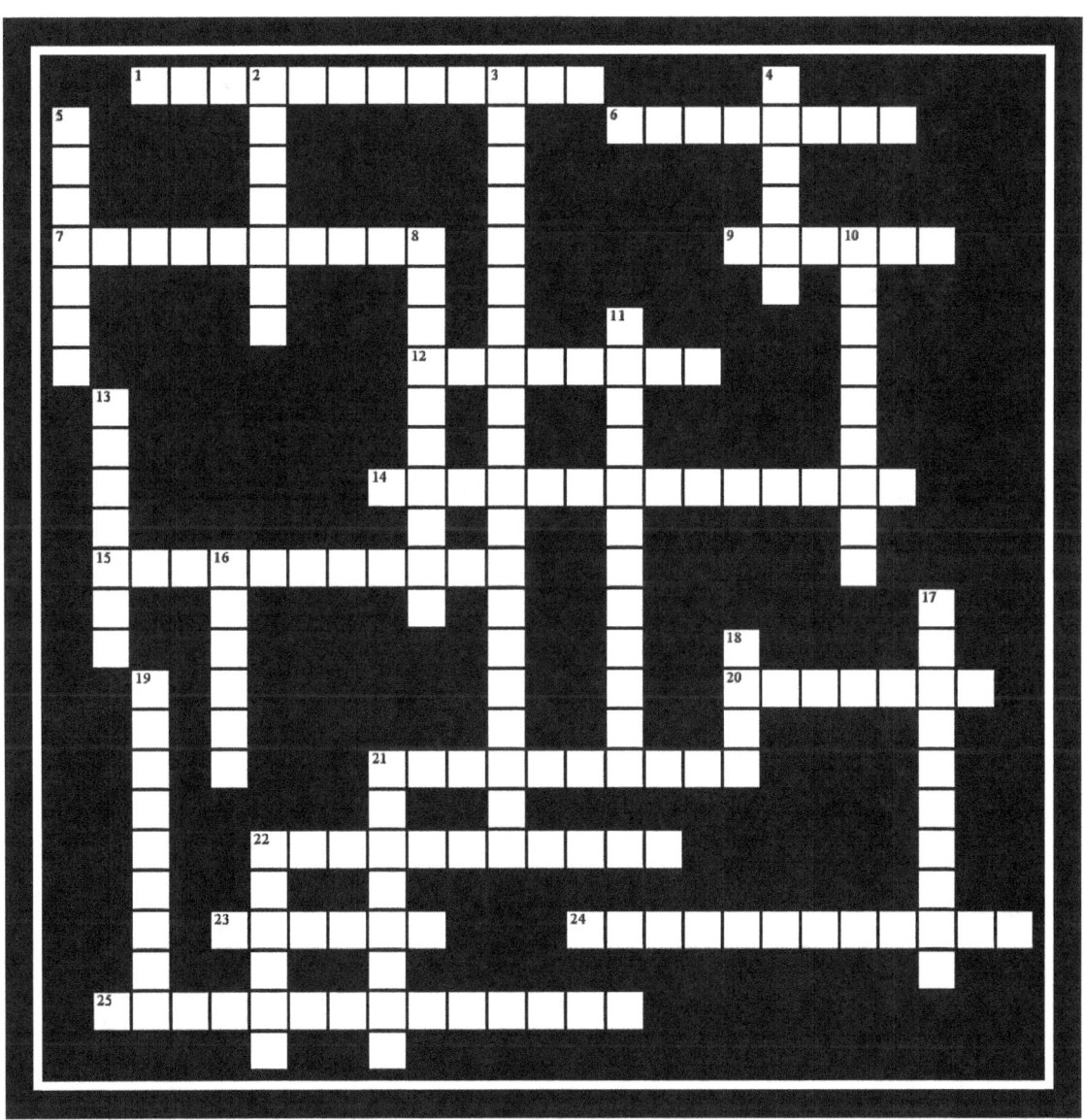

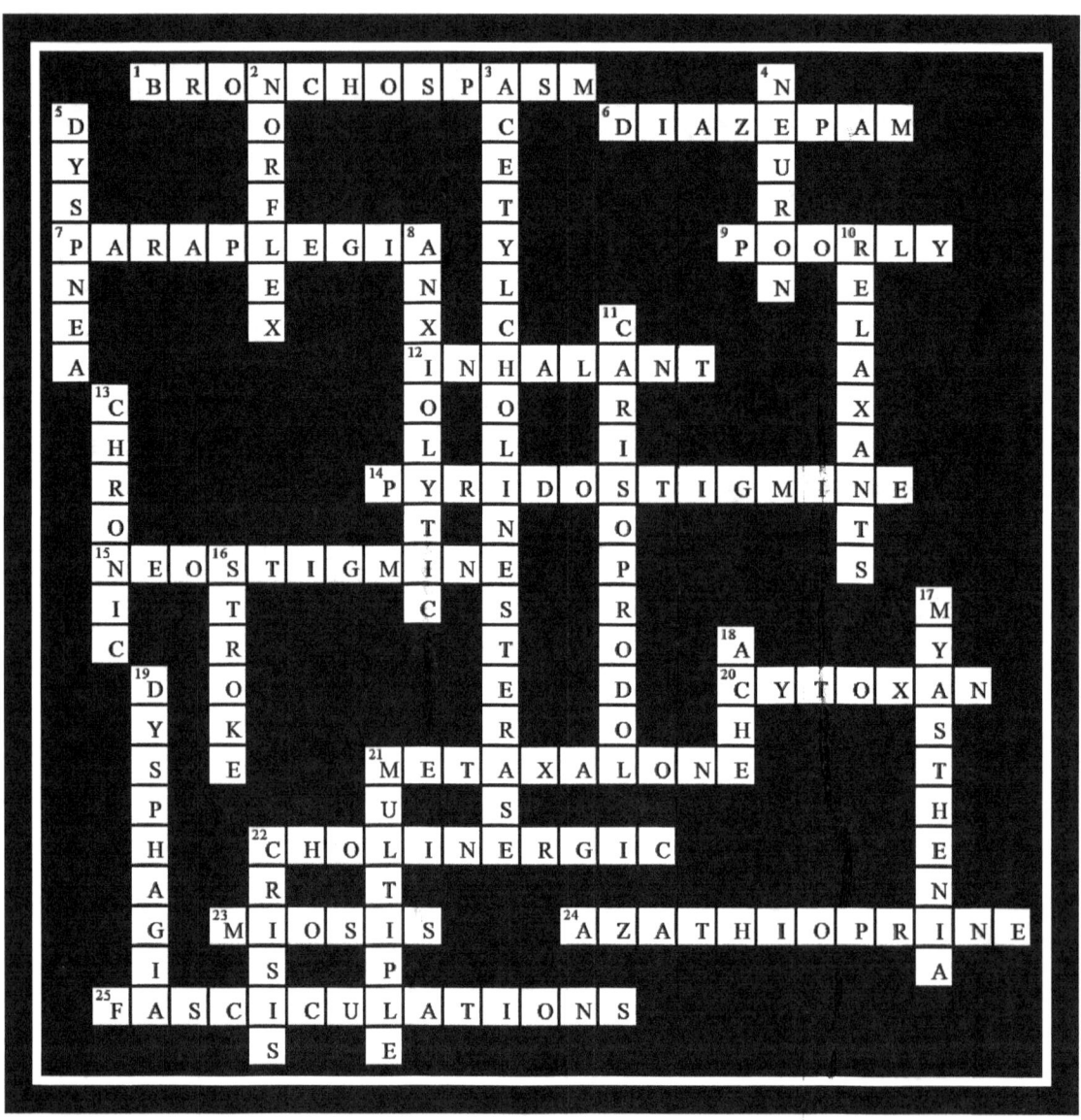

Pharmacology
Crossword Challenge
Neurologic & Neuromuscular Agents
Neuromuscular Disorders
Section V
Notes

Across

2. These are sensory pain receptors activated by noxious stimuli in peripheral tissues.
5. The generic name for Ultram. Contraindicated in severe alcoholism or with use of opioids.
6. This opioid antagonist is an antidote for morphine overdose.
13. These drugs treat moderate-to-severe rheumatoid arthritis by disrupting the inflammatory process.
15. A commonly used abbreviation for "disease-modifying antirheumatic drug."
17. The generic name for Demerol.
18. This adverse reaction is typically caused by taking aspirin.
19. This drug is the best choice when treating an acute gout attack.
20. This is not an antiinflammatory. It inhibits the final steps of uric acid biosynthesis. Used as a prophylactic to prevent gout.
23. Opioid analgesics are called opioid ___.
26. Chemical mediators. Causes vasodilation and relaxation of smooth muscle.
28. Another term for gold drug therapy.
29. The first mediator in the inflammatory process.

Down

1. The most commonly used abbreviation for "patient-controlled analgesia."
3. Second-generation NSAIDs. Selective ___ inhibitors.
4. These drugs increase the rate of uric acid excretion by inhibiting its reabsorption.
7. Medications that have been developed for other purposes and later found to be effective for pain relief in neuropathy are known as ___ analgesics.
8. This type of pain is an unusual sensory disturbance often involving neural supersensitivity.
9. This syndrome is caused by physical dependence.
10. These agents are used to treat refractory rheumatory arthritis.
11. An extraction from opium, this drug is a potent opioid analgesic.
12. The five responses to tissue injury are called the ___ signs of inflammation.
14. The generic name for Duragesic.
16. For the patient receiving periodic morphine IV push, it is critical to monitor ___.
21. A reaction to tissue injury caused by the release of chemical mediators.
22. This type of opioid analgesic provides a continuous "around-the-clock" pain control that is helpful to patients who suffer from chronic pain.
23. A psychologic and physical dependence upon a substance beyond normal voluntary control.
24. Caused by microorganisms and results in inflammation.
25. The most commonly used abbreviation for nonsteroid antiinflammatory drug.
27. The "disease of kings."

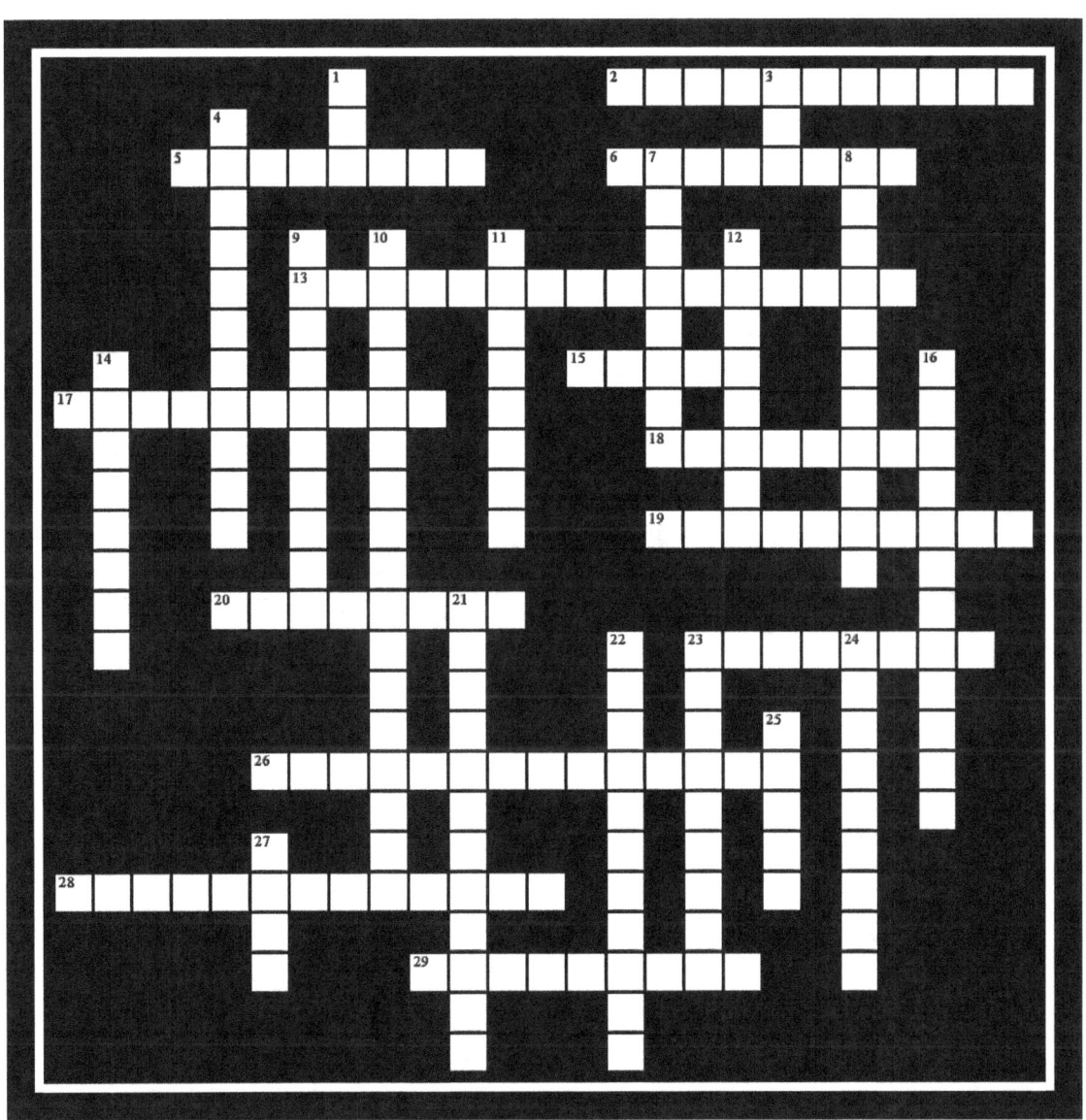

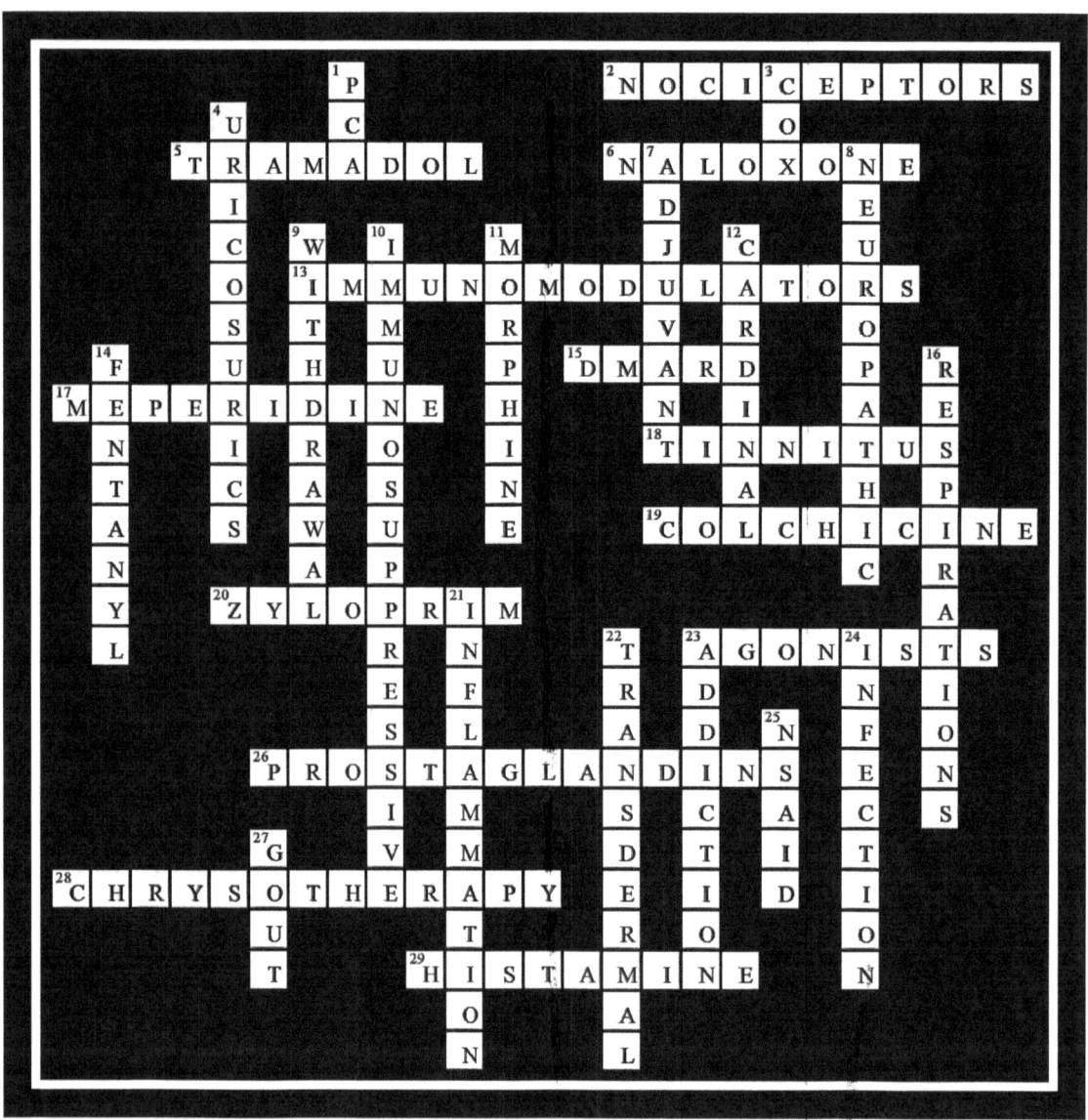

Pharmacology
Crossword Challenge
Pain & Inflammation
Section VI
Notes

Across

1. This drug may cause confusion and blurred vision.
6. This phenothiazine produces a strong sedative effect and decreased blood pressure.
8. This drug alters the effects of dopamine by blocking dopamine receptors. Sedation and EPS may occur.
11. A trade name for lorazepam.
14. Any drug that modifies psychotic behavior and exerts an antipsychotic effect.
15. This type of low blood pressure occurs when an individual assumes an upright position from a supine position. ___ hypotension.
16. This type of dyskinesia is a serious adverse reaction occurring in clients who have taken a typical antipsychotic drug for more than a year.
21. Neuroleptics or psychotropics.
23. The generic term for Cogentin. Used to treat extrapyramidal symptoms.
24. The generic term for Clozaril.
26. A syndrome characterized by an inability to remain in a sitting posture, with motor restlessness and a feeling of muscular quivering; may appear as a side effect of antipsychotic and neuroleptic medication.
27. This anxiolytic is used in the management of anxiety and alcohol withdrawal.

Down

2. An agent that prevents or relieves nausea and vomiting.
3. This phenothiazine has a strong sedative effect, causes few EPS and has no antiemetic effects.
4. This phenothiazine produces a low sedative and strong antiemetic effect and may have little effect on blood pressure.
5. This group of agents is part of the nonphenothiazine group.
7. Antipsychotics act by blocking action of ___.
9. A condition whereby there is a loss of contact with reality.
10. Benzodiazepines cause anxiety to ___.
12. The GABA neurotransmitter is associated with the regulation of ___.
13. The generic term for Moban.
17. The most common side effect for all antipsychotics.
18. Facial grimacing, involuntary upward eye movement, muscle spasms of the tongue and face are indicative of acute ___.
19. The generic name for Mellaril.
20. Blood cell disorders.
22. A trade name for fluphenazine.
23. The mode of action for fluphenazine is to ___ dopamine receptors in the brain and control psychotic symptoms.
25. The commonly used abbreviation for Gamma-aminobutyric acid.

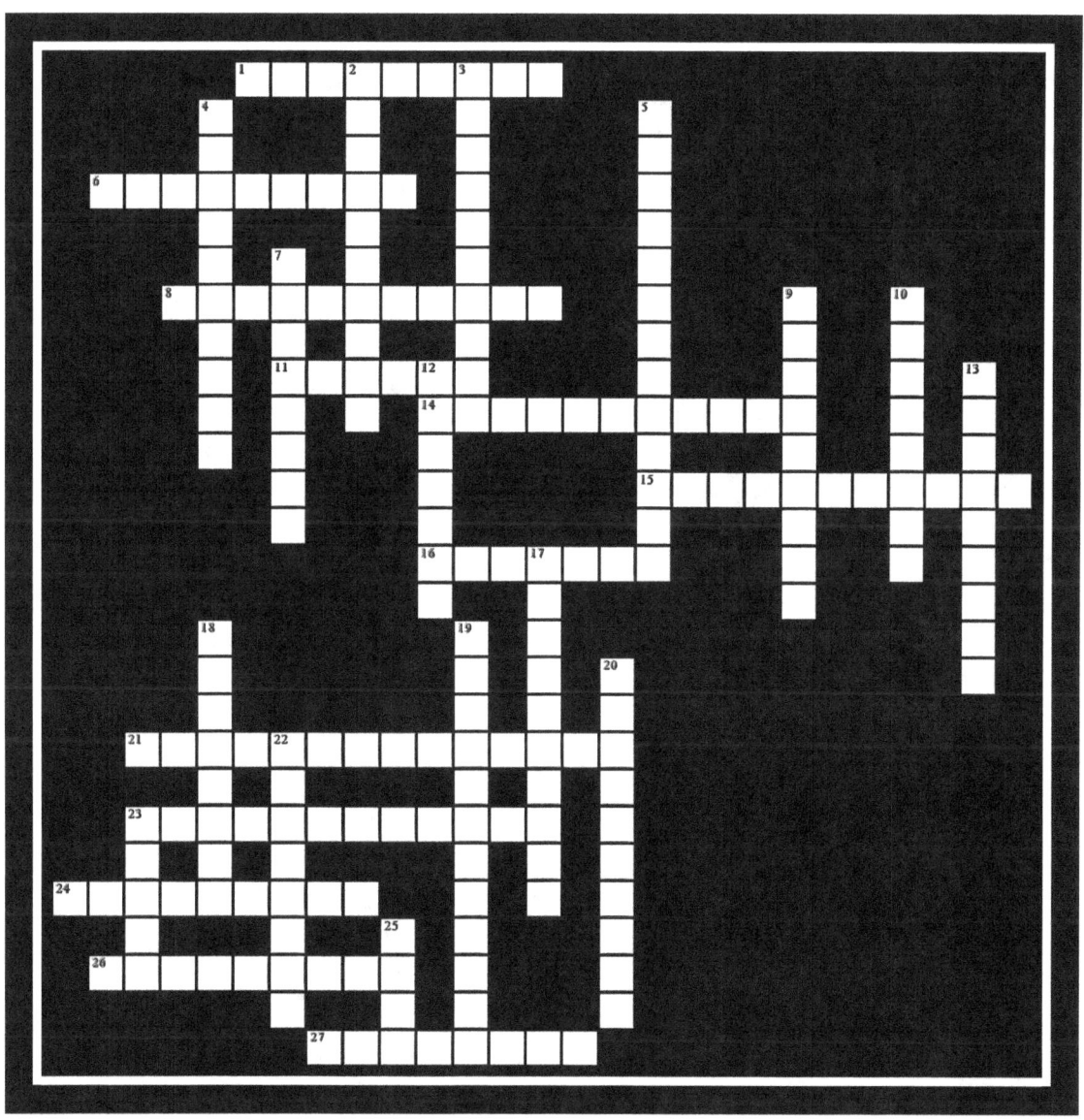

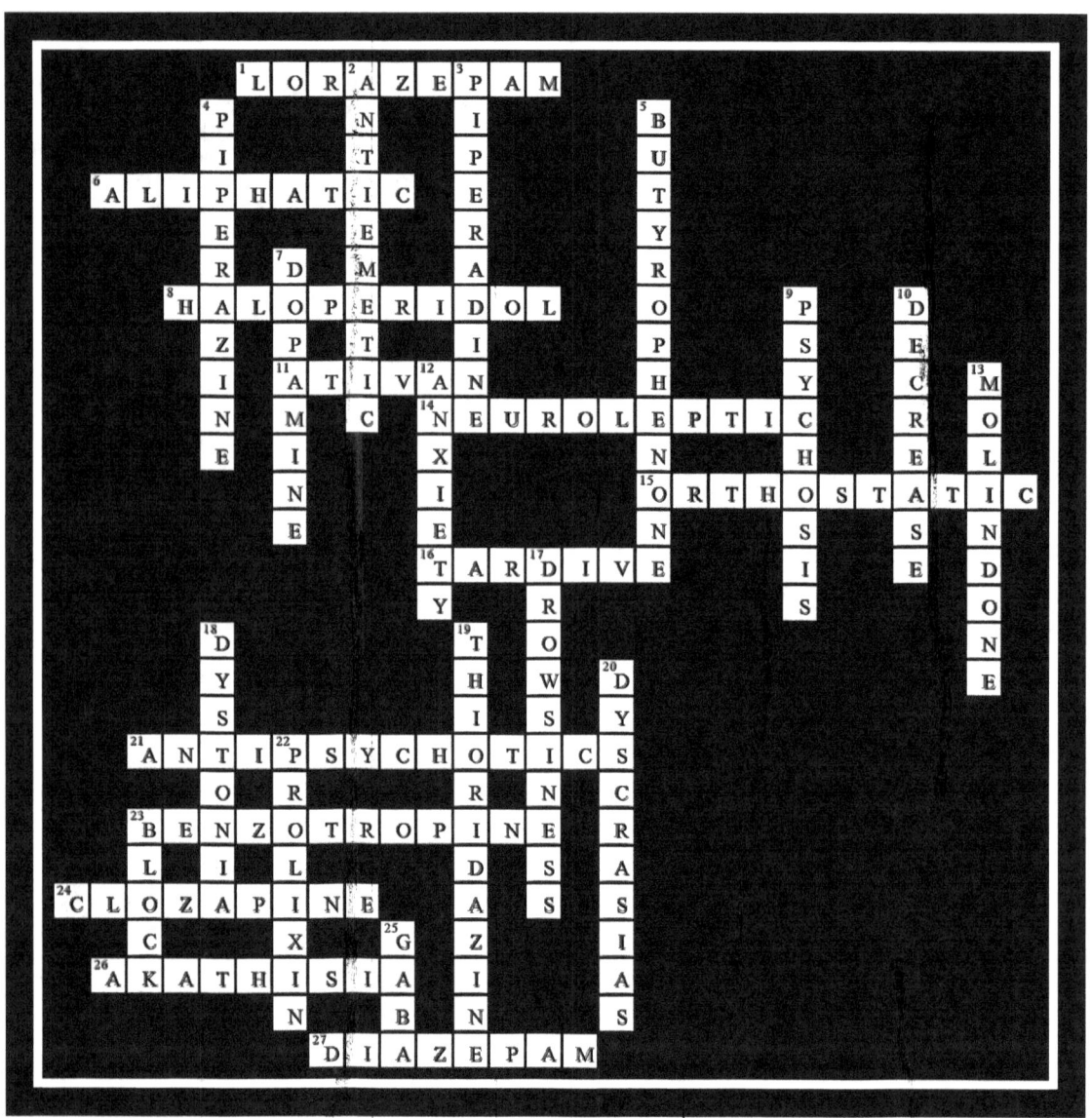

Pharmacology
Crossword Challenge
Psychiatric Agents
Antipsychotics & Anxiolytics
Section VII
Notes

Pharmacology
Crossword Challenge
Psychiatric Agents
Antidepressants & Mood Stabilizers
Section VII

Across

3. Fluoxetine is metabolized and excreted by the ___ .

5. A trade name for paroxetine. May be used for treatment of OCD.

9. Concurrent NSAIDs may cause lithium levels to ___ .

11. This drug is approved to treat acute mania.

13. This type of depression usually has a sudden onset after a precipitating event; e.g., depression resulting from a loss such as a death of a loved one.

14. The first TCA marketed in the 1950s.

16. A trade name for selegiline. An MAOI used in the treatment of major depression.

19. Generic name for Lamictal.

22. The enzyme monoamine oxidase ___ norepinephrine, dopamine, epinephrine and serotonin.

23. Trade name for carbamazepine, has been used in place of lithium for some patients.

25. Lithium tends to deplete ___ .

26. The generic name for Zoloft. The most commonly prescribed antidepressant.

28. The most commonly used abbreviation for selective serotonin reuptake inhibitor.

Down

1. An adverse reaction which may occur in patients taking Prozac.

2. Commonly used abbreviation for monoamine oxidase inhibitor.

4. This drug is used to treat bipolar affective disorder for some patients in place of lithium.

6. The generic term for Elavil. Antidepressant.

7. This drug was the first drug used to manage bipolar affective disorder.

8. Antidepressants can ___ suicidal tendencies.

10. Atypical antidepressants, second-generation antidepressants, used for major depression, reactive depression and anxiety.

12. another term for mood elevators.

15. The generic term for Prozac.

17. The term used to describe major depression characterized by loss of interest in work and home, inability to complete tasks and deep depression.

18. This may be a severe side effect for patients taking Sinequan.

20. The most common psychiatric problem affecting approximately 10%-20% of the population.

21. This drug is an example of an SSRI.

24. The commonly used abbreviation for tricyclic antidepressant.

27. The abbreviation for electroconvulsive therapy.

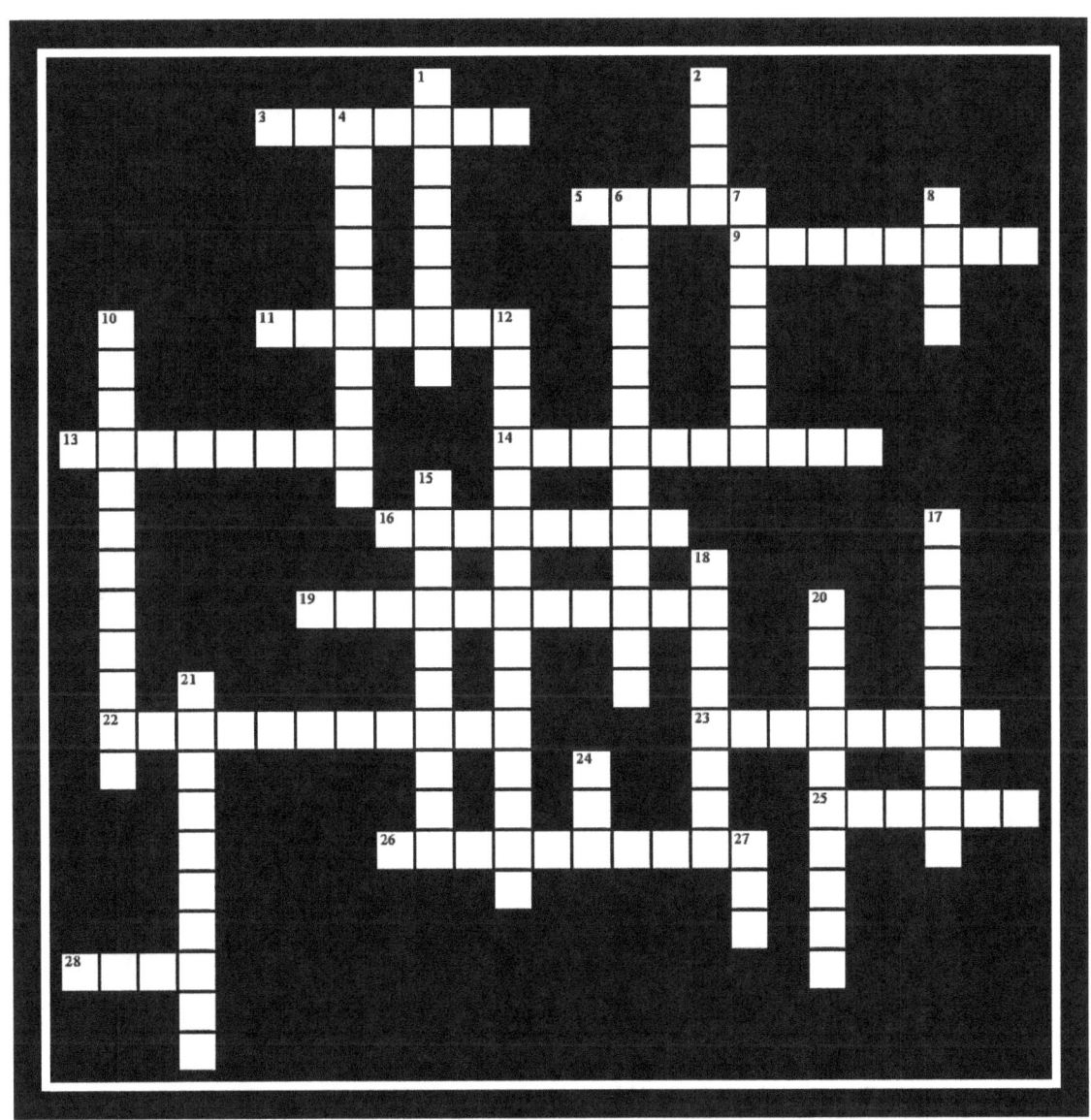

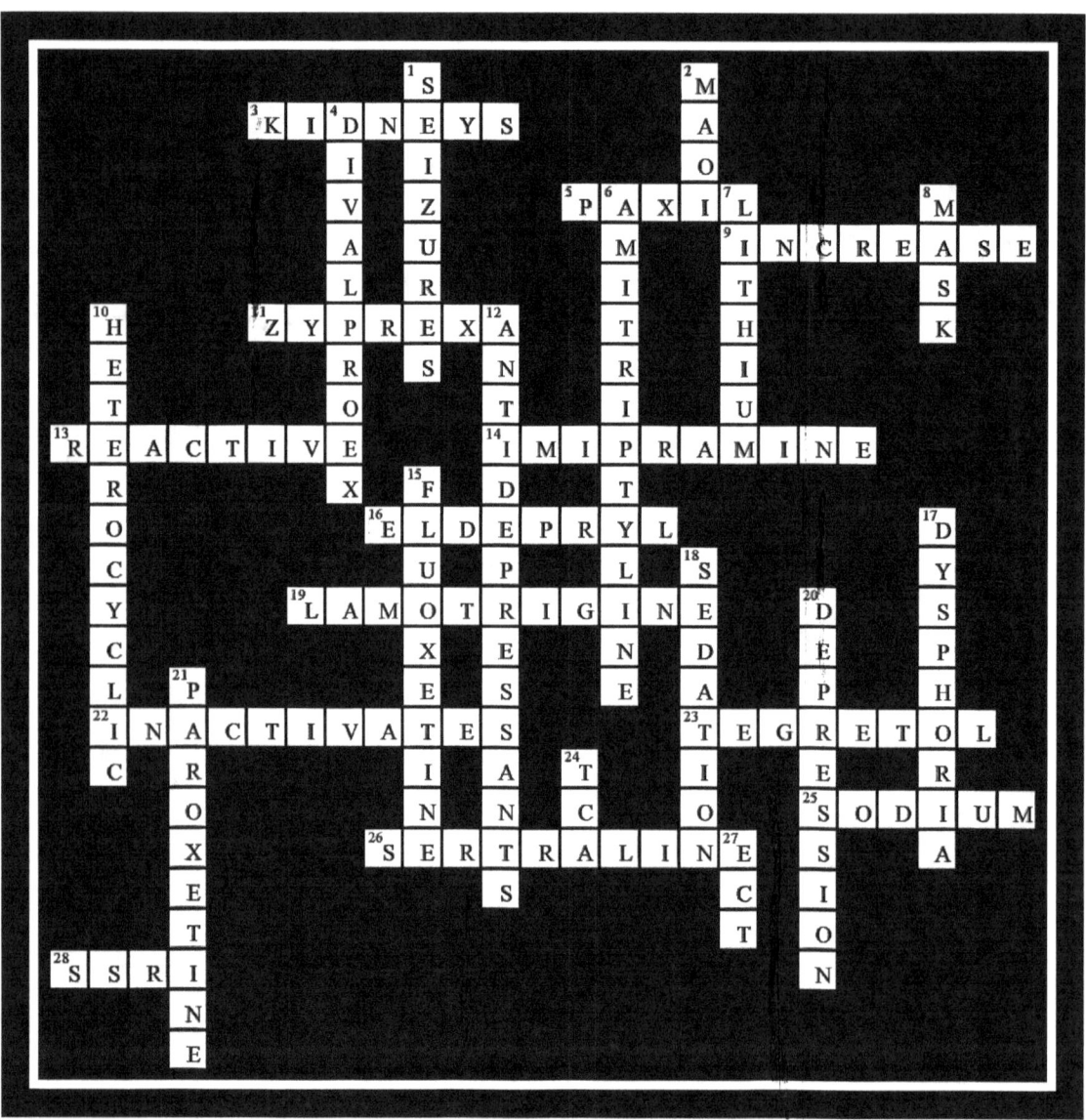

Pharmacology
Crossword Challenge
Psychiatric Agents
Antidepressants & Mood Stabilizers
Section VII
Notes

Across

1. Used to treat severe appendicitis, skin infections and pneumonia (piperacillin/tazobactam).
5. Azithromycin inhibits protein ___.
6. Beta-lactam structure. They inhibit the bacterial enzyme necessary for cell wall synthesis.
11. This type of resistance is caused by prior exposure to an antibacterial.
13. The generic term for Nafcin. Highly effective against penicillin G-resistant *Staphylococcus aureus.*
16. The generic name for penicillinase-resistant penicillin
19. Amoxicillin. The action of this drug is by ___ of bacterial cell-wall synthesis.
20. Cefadroxil is one of only a few cephalosporins which may be administered ___.
21. An adverse effect of taking lincosamides is pseudomembranous ___.
23. Another term for toxicity to the kidneys.
27. The generic term for Keflex.
29. This antibiotic is effective against MRSA, VRE and penicillin-resistant streptococci.
30. First broad-spectrum antibiotics effective against Gram-positive and Gram-negative bacteria.
31. Antibody proteins such as IgG and IgM. Elements of the immune response system.

Down

2. Occurrence of a secondary infection when the flora of the body is disturbed.
3. The shape of spirilla
4. Taking these agents can prevent absorption of tetracycline from the GI tract.
7. This enzyme produced by the microorganism is responsible for causing its penicillin resistance.
8. Frequently used as a preoperative bowel antiseptic.
9. A term used to describe damage to the auditory or vestibular branch of cranial nerve VIII.
10. Cefoperazone (Cefobid) is a ___-generation cephalosporin.
12. Another term used to describe disease-producing microorganisms.
14. Antibacterials. Substances that inhibit bacterial growth or kill bacteria and other microorganisms.
15. These agents inhibit the growth of bacteria.
17. Side effects, adverse reactions of penicillins include ___anemia.
18. These agents kill bacteria.
21. The shape of this bacteria is spherical.
22. Cefaclor (Ceclor) is used to treat ___infections.
24. A classification of antibiotics structurally related to macrolides.
25. These bacteria are elongated in shape.
26. The generic term for Omnicef.
28. Penicillin V potassium is not recommended for patients in ___ failure.

Pharmacology
Crossword Challenge
Antibacterial Agents
Antibacterials
Section VIII

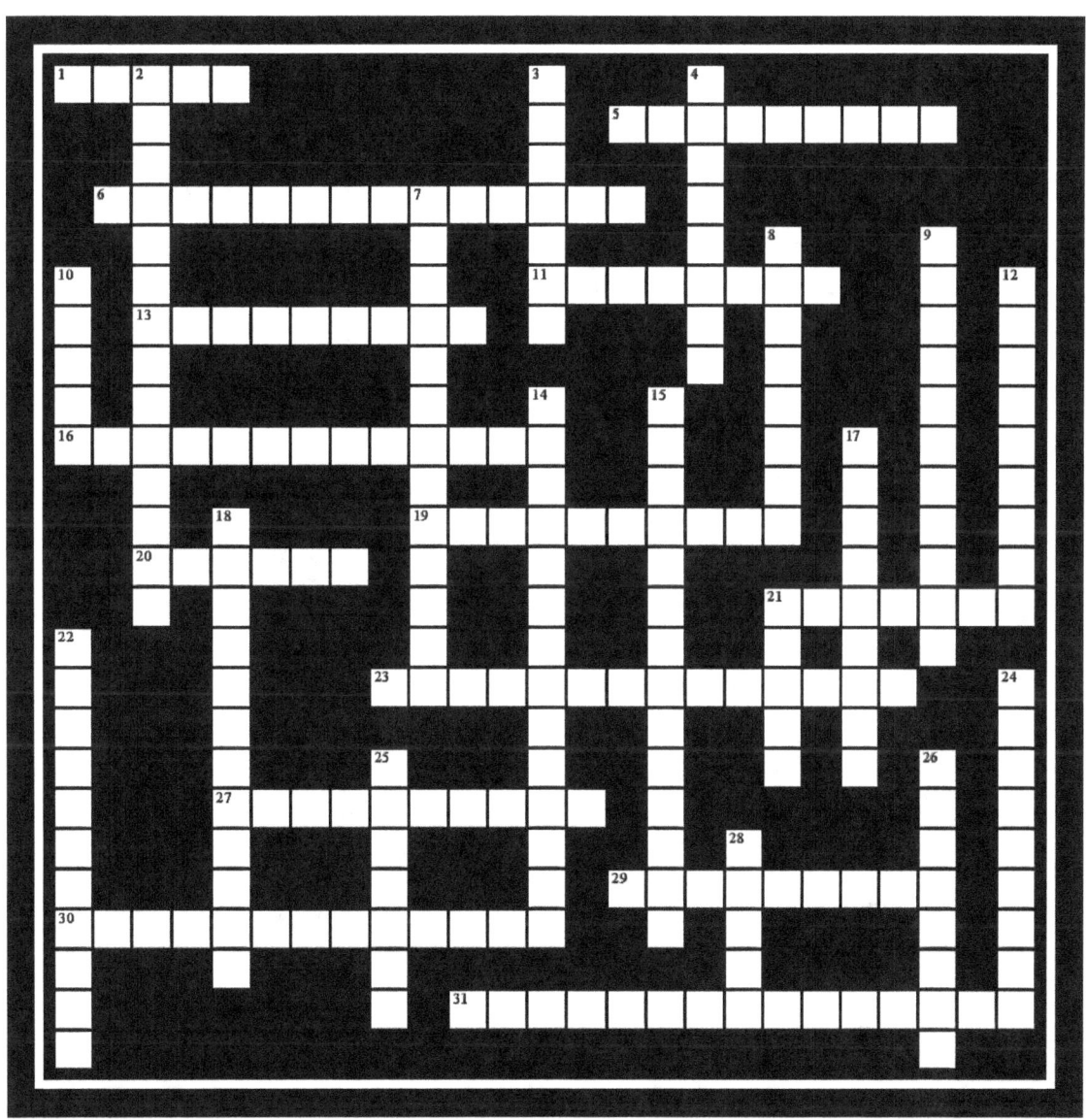

Pharmacology
Crossword Challenge
Antibacterial Agents
Antibacterials
Section VIII

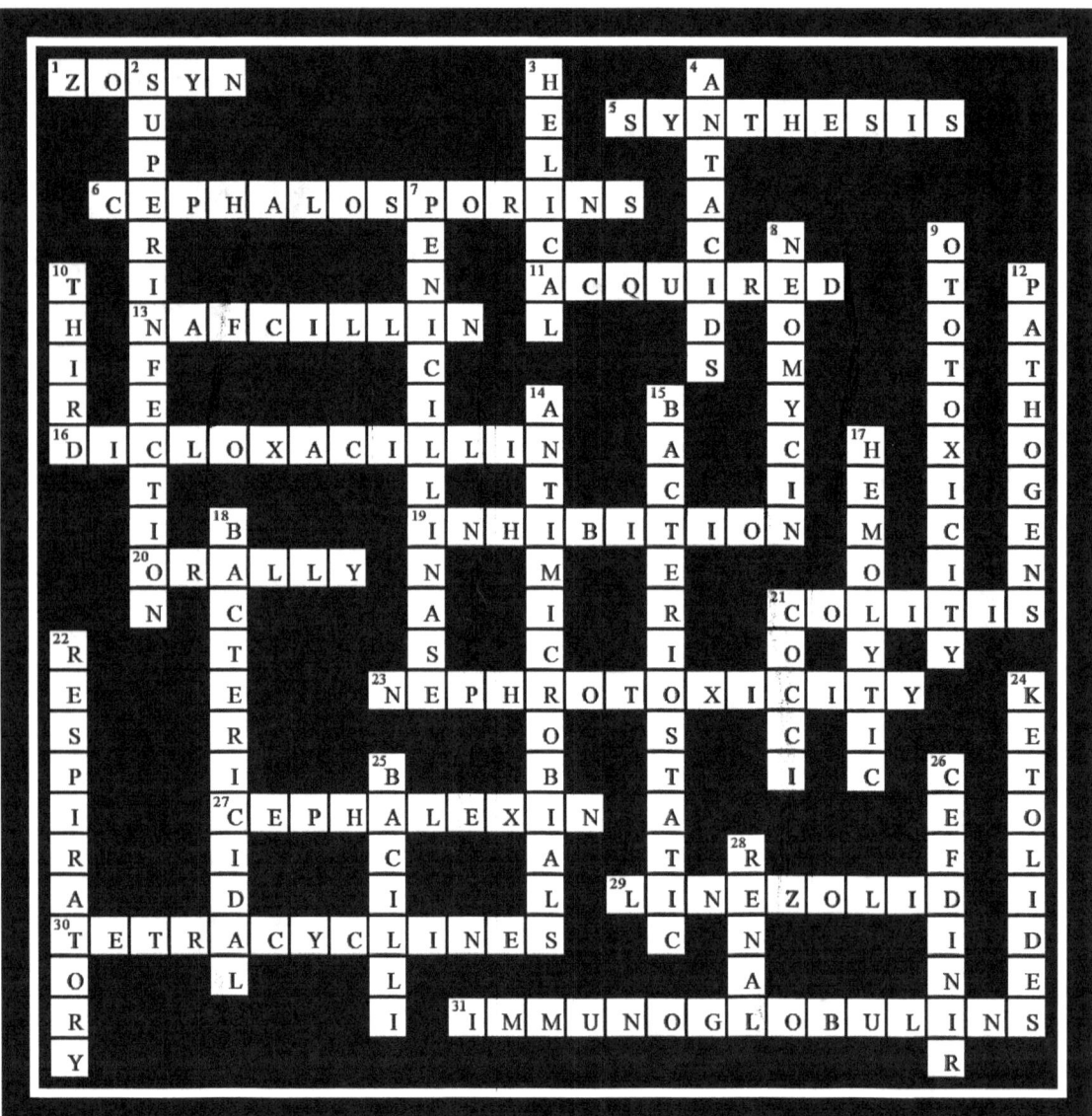

Pharmacology
Crossword Challenge
Antibacterial Agents
Antibacterials
Section VIII
Notes

Pharmacology
Crossword Challenge
Antibacterial Agents
Sulfonamide & Anti-infective Agents
Section VIII

Across

4. This type of effect is a coordinated or correlated action of two or more structures, agents, or physiologic processes so that the combined action is greater than the sum of each acting separately.

5. Also called antifungal, these are drugs used to treat fungal infections.

8. A trade name for metronidazole.

9. Sulfonamides are considered ___ because they inhibit bacterial synthesis of folic acid.

12. This drug is part of the azole group and used to treat systemic fungal infection.

13. These organisms are divided into yeasts and molds.

15. Avoid sulfonamides during the ___ trimester of pregnancy.

16. Erythematous macular, papular or vesicular eruption, erythema ___.

19. This polyene antifungal drug is used for treating severe system infection.

24. A common adverse reaction to isoniazid is ___.

25. The generic term for Gantrisin, a short-acting sulfonamide.

26. Patients taking this herb may develop hepatotoxicity if given ketoconazole.

27. The action of this group is to inhibit biosynthesis of essential components of the fungal cell wall which interferes with growth and reproduction.

Down

1. The patient should not drink this when taking metronidazole.

2. Trade name for voriconazole.

3. Polymyxin and bacitracin are in the group of ___.

6. This yeast is resistant to penicillin-type antibiotics and a common cause of infection of the mucous membranes.

7. A term used to describe crystals in the urine.

10. This group of drugs act by disrupting mitochondrial electron transport and inhibiting DNA synthesis.

11. This is a type of sensitivity or allergy to one sulfonamide that may lead to sensitivity to another sulfonamide.

14. This type of dermatitis causes desquamation, scaling and itching of the skin.

15. This antibacterial agent interferes with bacterial folic acid synthesis just as sulfonamides do.

17. An appropriate treatment for vaginal candidiasis.

18. Sulfonamides are not classified as an antibiotic because they were not obtained from these substances.

20. The generic name for Mycostatin. Administered orally or topically to treat candidal infection.

21. Sulfonamides are most effective against Escherichia coli and ___.

22. Patients taking amphotericin B should be aware of this sign or symptom.

23. A topical sulfonamide used to treat burns.

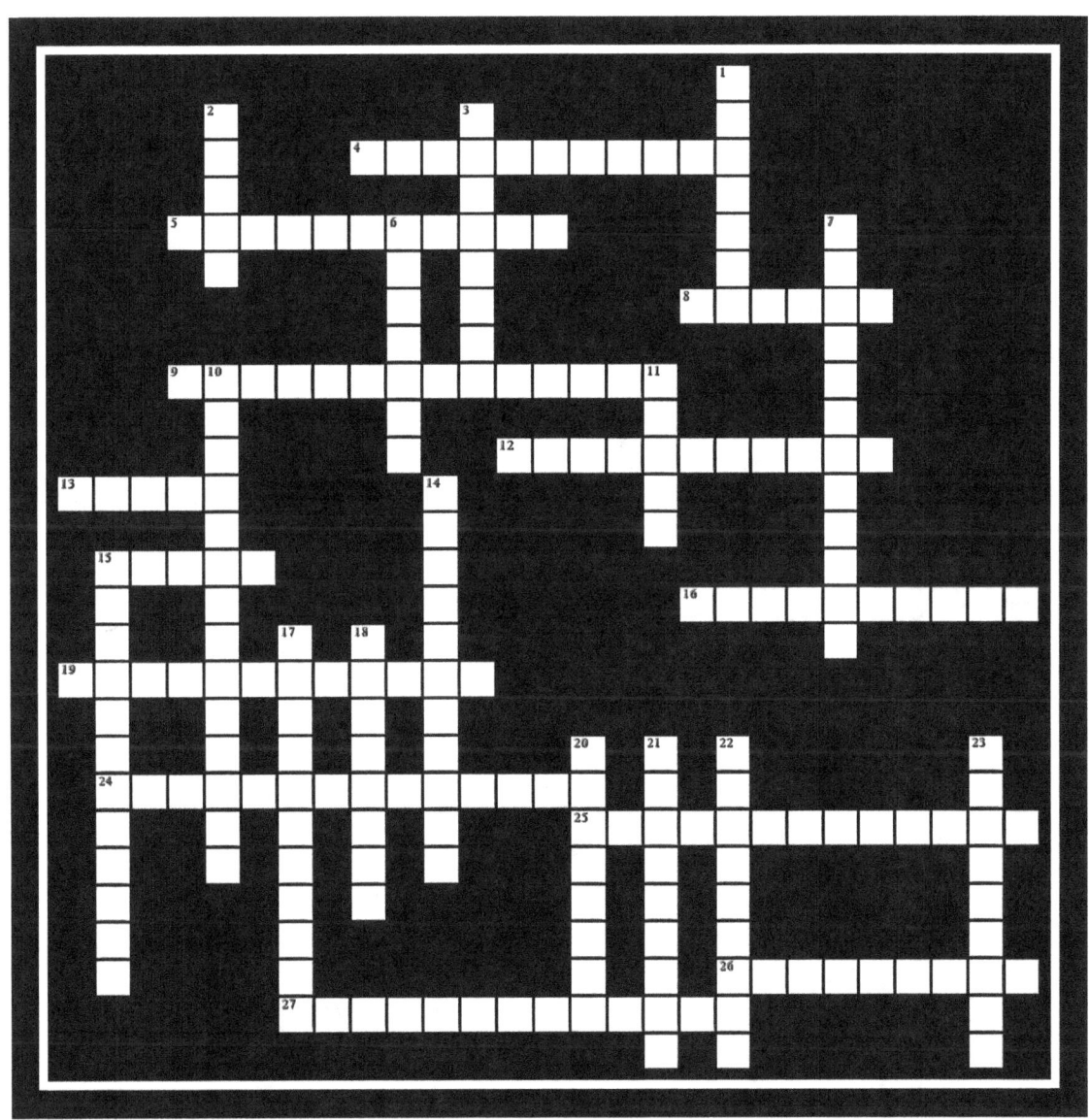

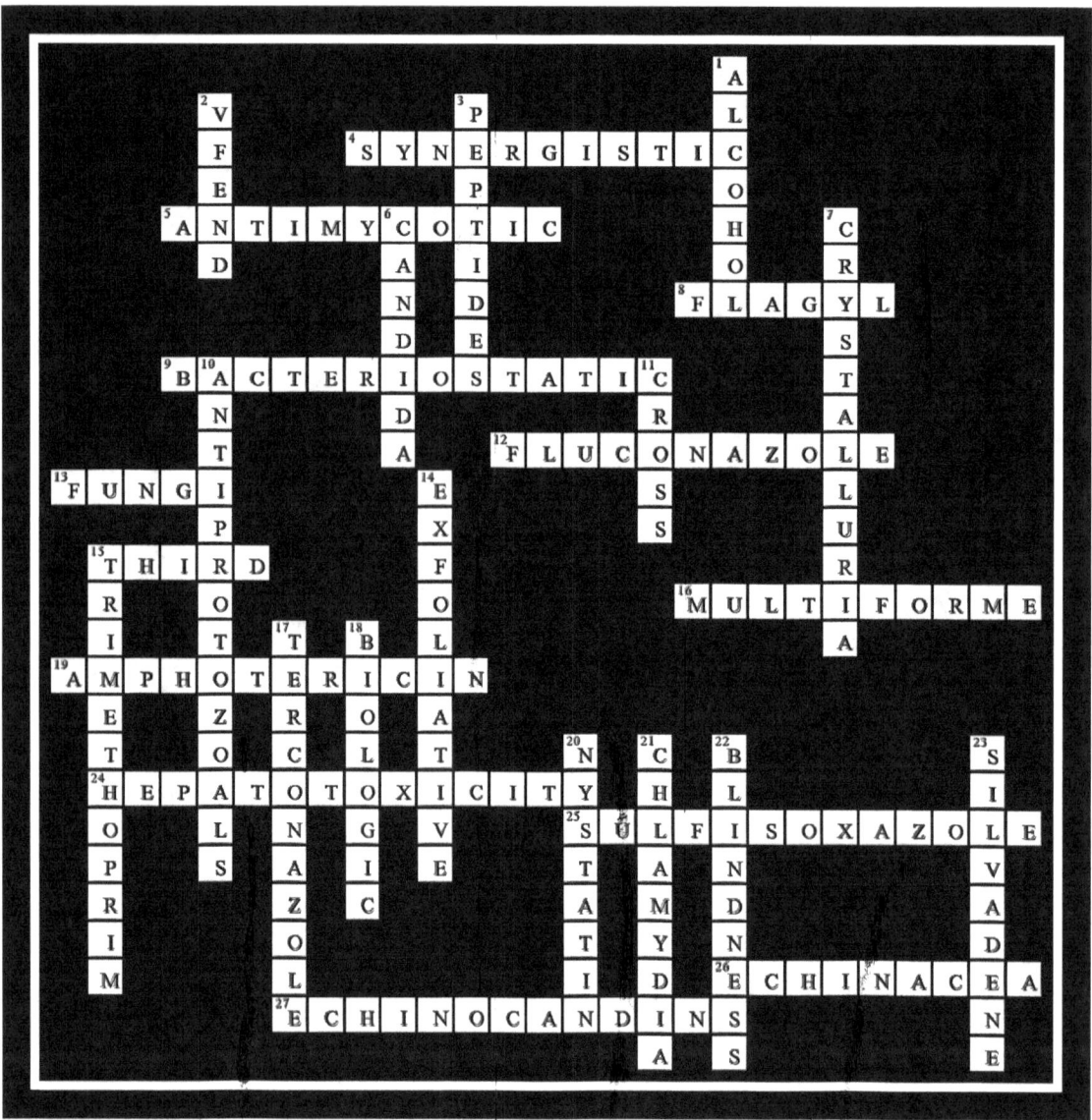

Pharmacology
Crossword Challenge
Antibacterial Agents
Sulfonamide & Anti-infective Agents
Section VIII
Notes

Pharmacology
Crossword Challenge
Immunologic Agents
HIV, AIDS & Vaccines
Section IX

Across

3. This opportunistic sarcoma causes dark blue lesions and usually appears early in the course of HIV.
6. Protection against infectious diseases.
7. The generic name for AZT. Its mode of action inhibits viral enzyme reverse transcriptase.
9. This is the correct route of administration for rotavirus vaccine.
11. Abbreviation for nonnucleoside reverse transcriptase inhibitor.
13. A biologic weapon, highly lethal.
15. Salmonella enterica typhi.
16. This is an acquired typed of immunity which develops in response to immunizations.
17. Immune system cells originate in the ___ (two words).
20. There are two broad categories of immunity: Acquired and ___.
24. The acquisition of detectable levels of antibodies in the bloodstream.
27. These types of medications are designed to slow or inhibit the HIV-related enzymes.
28. This is the last of 10 steps in HIV replication of the HIV life cycle.
29. Trade name Kaletra. Its mode of action is to inhibit HIV protease, rendering enzyme incapable of processing polyprotease precursors.

Down

1. Trade name Epivir. This drug is a member of the NRTI category.
2. This condition is contraindicated for the use of the varicella vaccine.
4. This type of inhibitor blocks the insertion of HIV DNA into human DNA by attacking the enzyme that allows them to merge.
5. Attenuated virus vaccines contain this type of microorganism.
8. Inactivated toxins.
10. To carry out the therapeutic plan.
12. HIV is considered this type of virus.
14. A commonly used abbreviation for highly active antiretroviral therapy.
18. Trade name Norvir. This drug is a member of the NNRTI category.
19. This pathogen is capable of causing disease only in a host whose resistance is lowered, e.g., by other diseases or by drugs.
21. Immunoglobulins.
22. This is one of the three types of inhibitors that make up the classification of drugs known as antiretroviral therapy.
23. Any substance that induces a state of sensitivity and/or immune response after a latent period.
25. Trade name Varivax. Used in the prevention of chickenpox.
26. This disease produces swelling of the salivary glands, fever and headache.

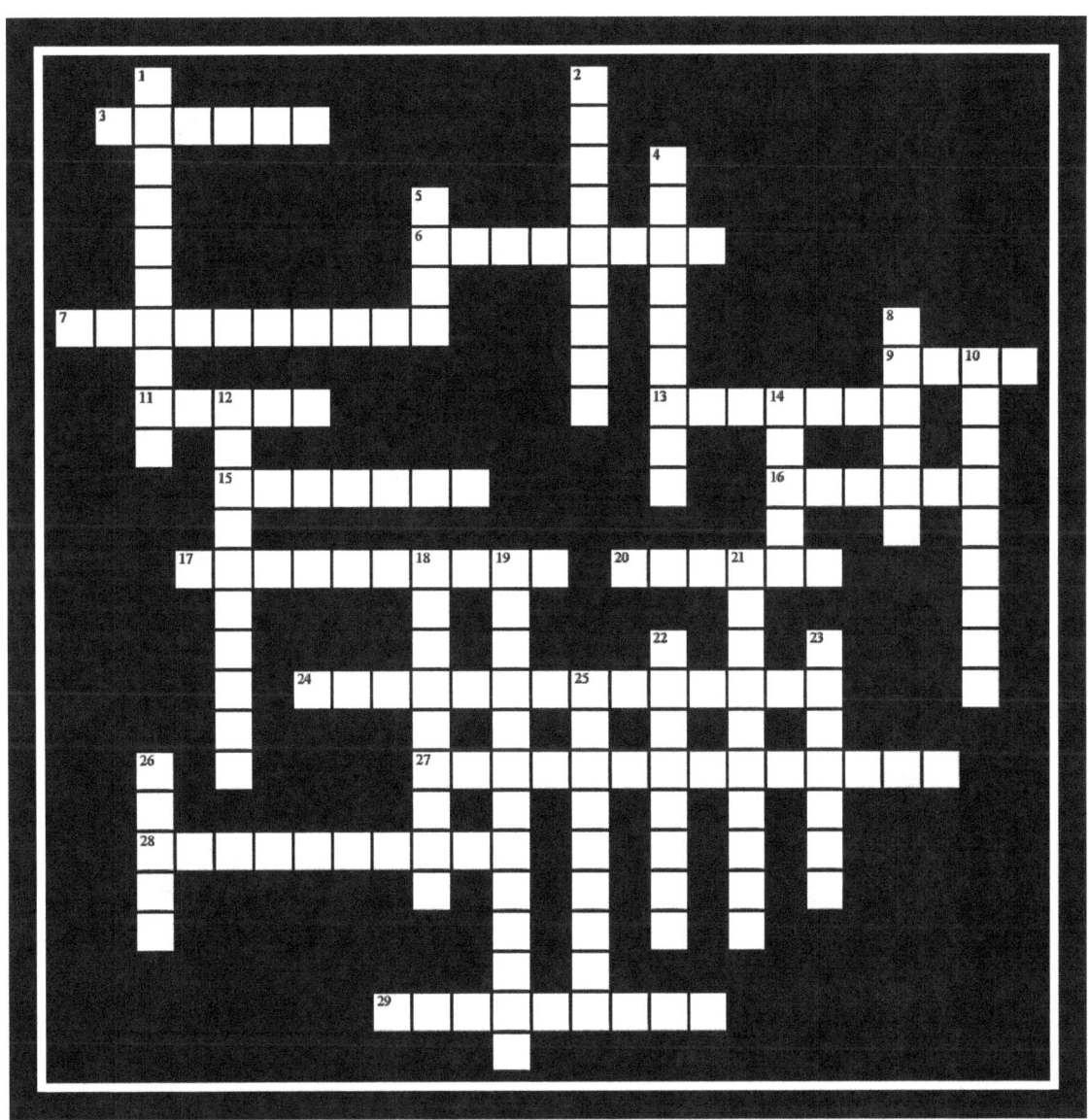

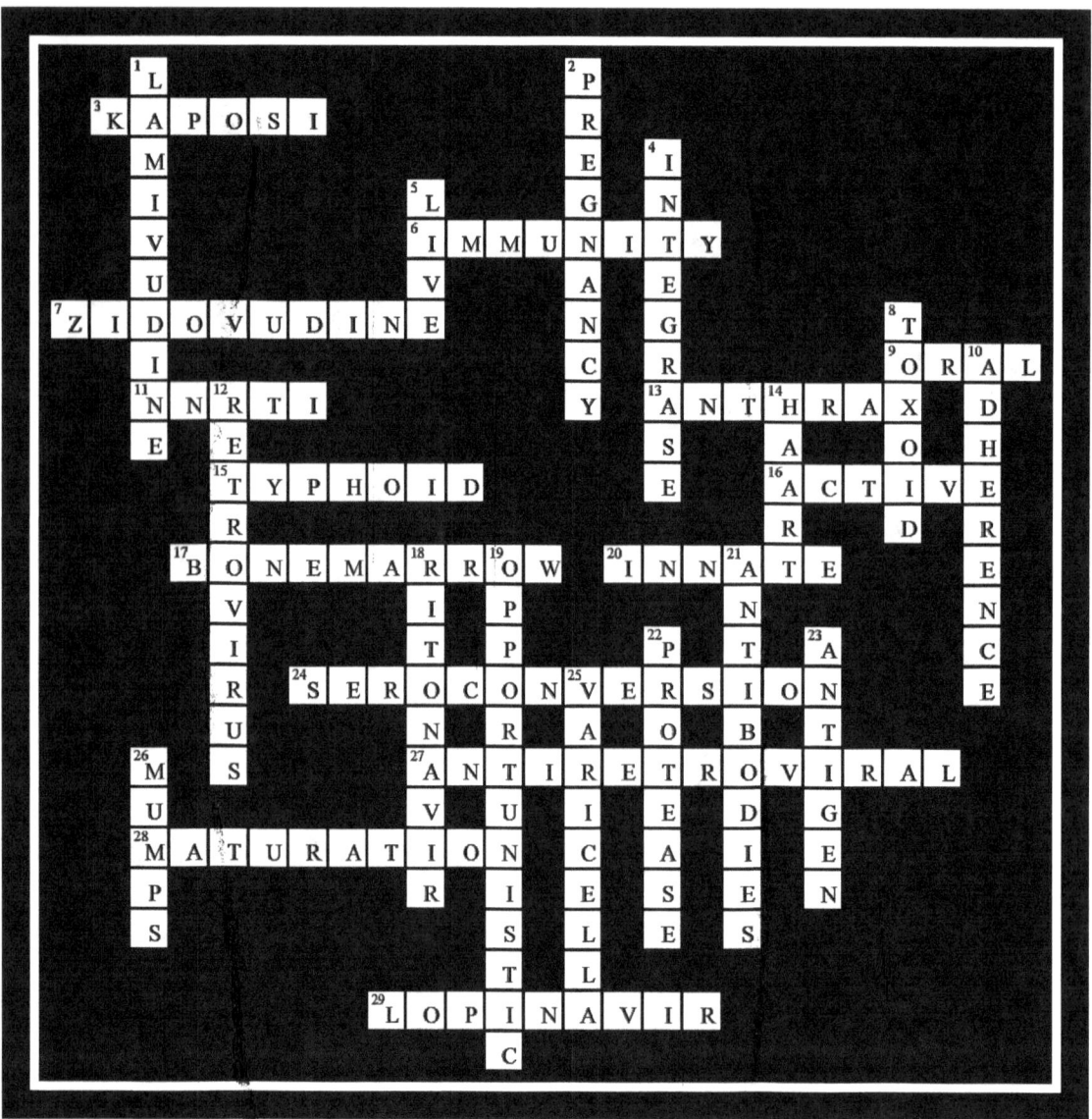

Pharmacology
Crossword Challenge
Immunologic Agents
HIV, AIDS & Vaccines
Section IX
Notes

Across

4. These proteins regulate the intensity & duration of immune response.
7. This type of chemotherapy describes the use of two or more chemotherapy agents.
9. The time it takes for the number of cells in a neoplasm to double, with shorter doubling times implying more rapid growth.
11. This type of therapy augments the natural ability of the immune system.
15. This "rescue" saves normal cells from the adverse reaction of MTX.
16. A term used to describe hair loss.
17. Abbreviation for methotrexate.
18. This type of chemotherapy involves packaging of drugs inside synthetic fat globules.
19. This alkaloid is extracted from the periwinkle plant.
20. This type of therapy is used to relieve symptoms associated with advanced disease.
21. Male hormone that promotes regression of tumors.
22. Generic term for Oncovin. Mitotic inhibitor. Affects cells in the M phase.
23. Generic term for Eulexin, antiandrogen.

Down

1. This type of therapy is often used to destroy cancer cells.
2. These inhibitors are derived from natural products and block cell division at the M phase.
3. These agents cause cross-linking of DNA strands and abnormal base pairing to prevent cells from dividing.
5. These type of antibiotics inhibit protein and RNA synthesis and bind DNA causing fragmentation.
6. These resemble natural metabolites which recycle and breakdown organic compounds.
8. This type of drug, often given with high-dose cyclophosphamide, inactivates urotoxic metabolites.
10. The generic term for 5-FU, an antimetabolite.
12. The generic term for Cytoxan.
13. Another term for cell death.
14. The generic term for Idamycin, antitumor antibiotic.
17. Spread of disease to other areas of the body.

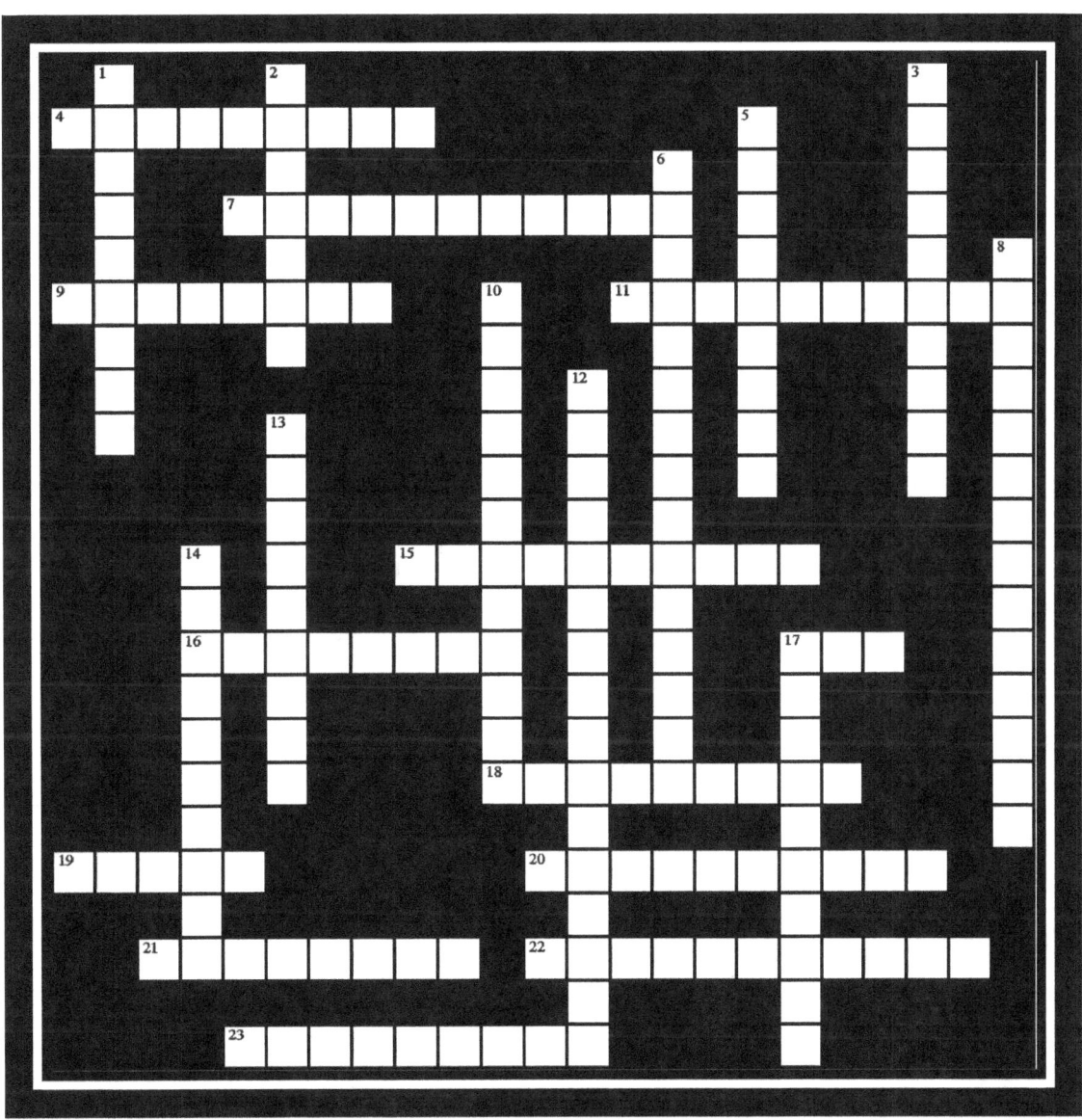

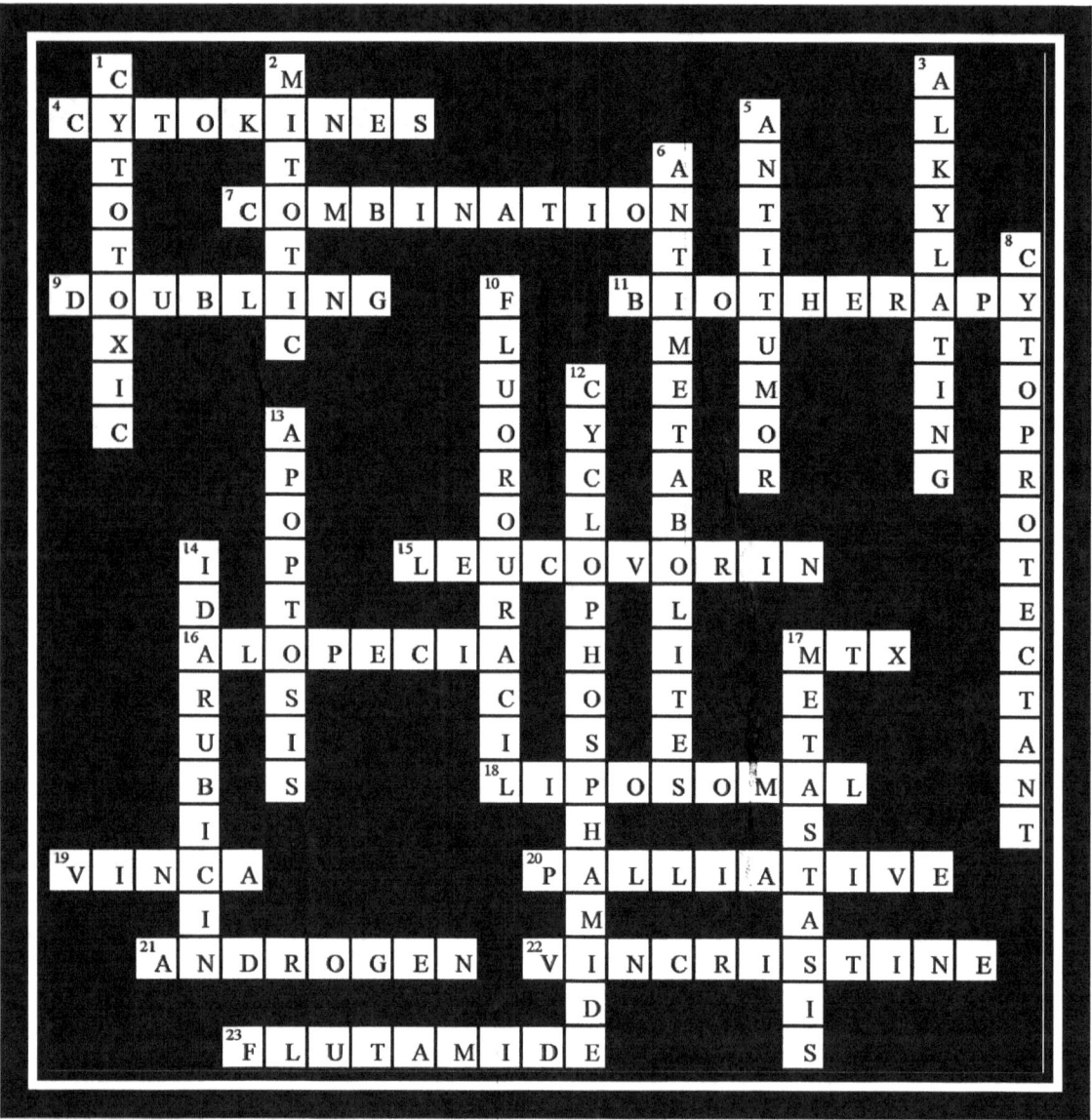

Pharmacology
Crossword Challenge
Antineoplastic Agents
Anticancer Drugs
Section X
Notes

Across

2. The generic term for Rituxan and is used to treat relapsed, low-grade NHL.

6. The commonly used abbreviation for protein tyrosine kinase.

8. The generic term for Velcade and is used in the treatment of multiple myeloma.

9. Intake of this CNS stimulant should be avoided by patients receiving targeted therapy.

12. This is the most important ligand involved in angiogenesis.

15. These antibodies, produced in the lab, are designed to bind to specific antigens on the surface of cancer cells.

17. Commonly used abbreviation for epidermal growth factor/receptor.

19. A common side effect for patient's taking Iressa.

20. This drug is an example of a topoisomerase II inhibitor. Used in treatment for small cell cancer of the lung.

21. Three types of engineered monoclonal antibodies include humanized, fully human antibodies and ___.

22. The generic term for Erbitux used in the treatment of metastatic colorectal cancer.

23. The generic term for Tarceva, used in treatment for locally advanced non-small cell lung cancer.

Down

1. Another term for a growth factor protein.

3. The cytochrome P450 systems are involved in drug metabolism and are known as ___.

4. The term used to describe cell death.

5. The generic term for Sutent, approved for advanced renal cell carcinoma.

7. This drug decreases the rate of drug metabolism which may increase toxicity for a patient on gefitinib.

10. A physiologic process of new capillary formation from existing blood vessels.

11. These inhibitors are nuclear enzymes that alter the shape of DNA coils.

13. The generic term for Avastin, an angiogenesis inhibitor.

14. The generic term for Nexavar, used in the treatment of metastatic renal cell cancer.

15. Commonly used abbreviation for mammalian target of rapamycin

16. The generic term for Camptosar, used in treatment for advanced carcinoma of colon and rectum.

18. These inhibitors are intracellular multienzyme complexes that degrade proteins.

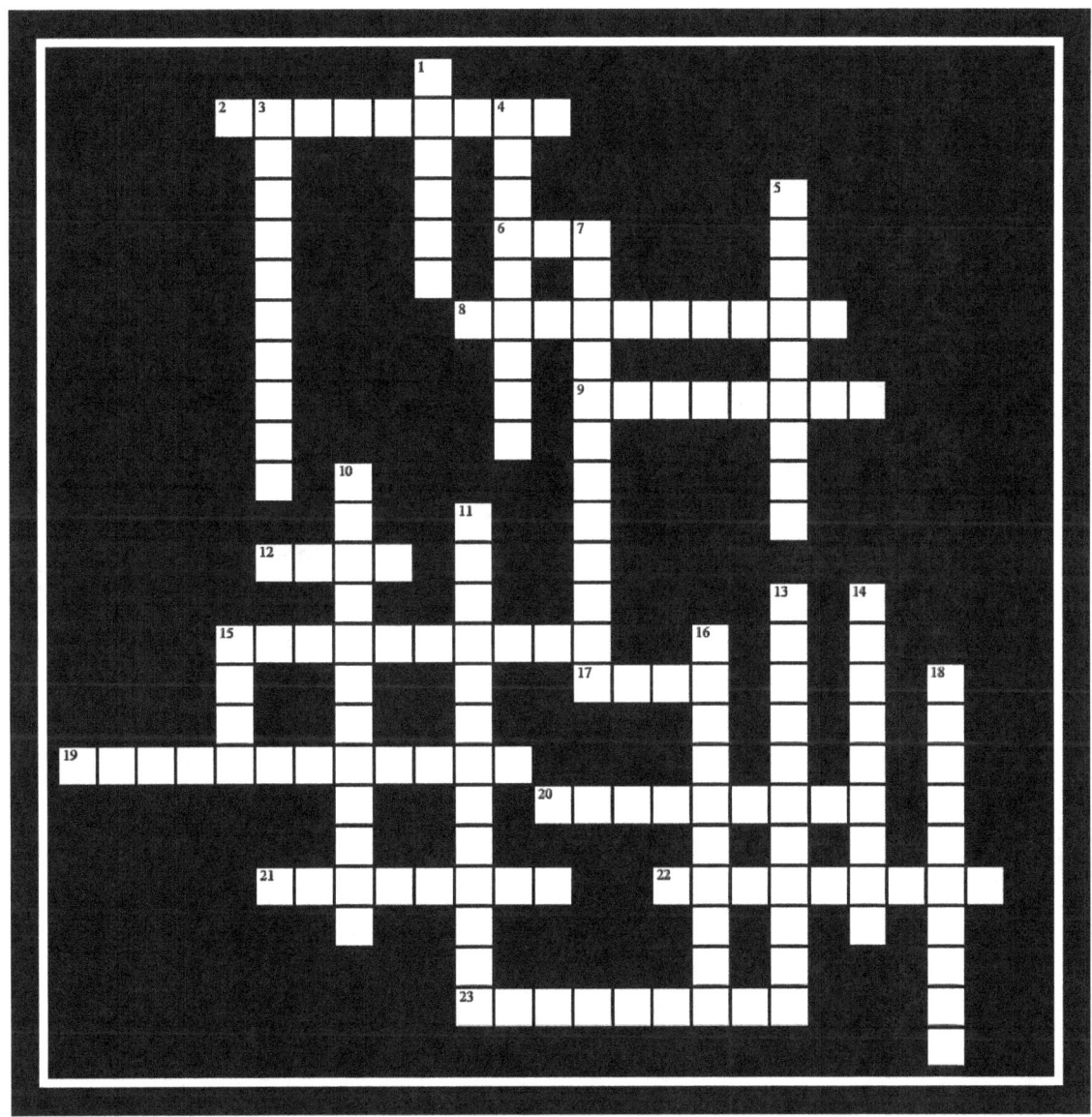

Pharmacology
Crossword Challenge
Antineoplastic Agents
Cancer Treatments
Section X

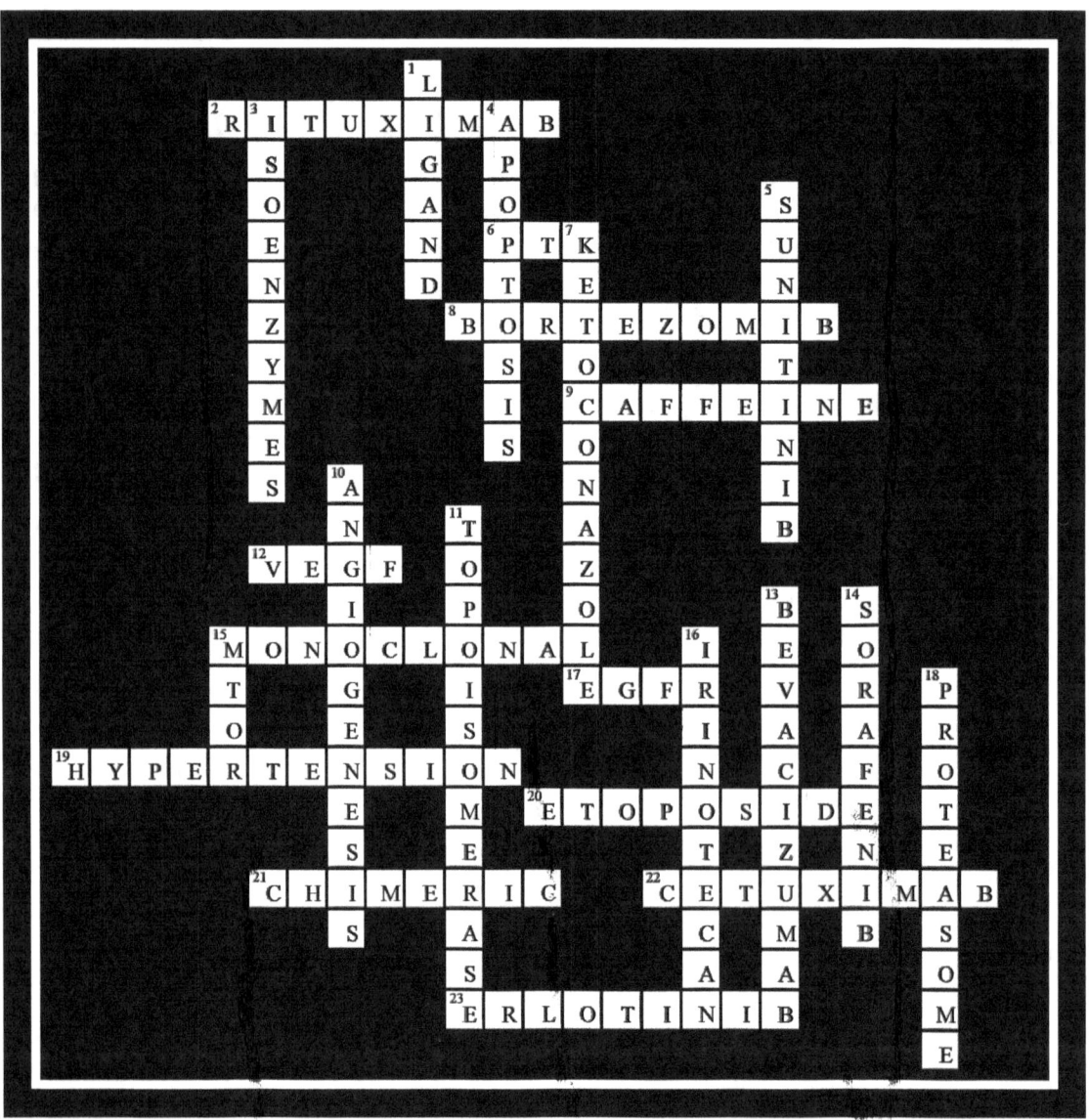

Pharmacology
Crossword Challenge
Antineoplastic Agents
Cancer Treatments
Section X
Notes

Across

1. Stimulates the formation of proerythroblasts & release of reticulocytes from bone marrow.
4. This type of DNA is the genetic engineering process that produces mass quantities of human protein.
5. The commonly used abbreviation for biologic response modifiers which is a class of pharmacologic agents used to enhance the body's immune system.
6. The commonly used abbreviation for granulocyte colony-stimulating factor.
10. A trade name for epoetin alfa.
13. Interferon ___ enhances the activity of suppressor T cells.
14. Suppression of bone marrow activity.
15. The commonly used abbreviation for epidermal growth factor receptor.
19. Overexpression of EGFR1 results in ___ cell proliferation.
20. The generic term for Leukine, increases production of eosinophils, macrophages, monocytes and neutrophils.
21. Erythropoietin is a glycoprotein produced by the ___.
23. This interleukin-2 is FDA-indicated for the treatment of metastatic renal cell carcinoma.
24. The major phagocytic cells of the immune system.

Down

2. A family of naturally occurring proteins.
3. A term used to describe a decreased number of thrombocytes in the blood.
6. G-CSF is a ___ produced by monocytes and fibroblasts.
7. Sargramostim ___ platelet production.
8. The lowest value of formed blood cells.
9. A type of white blood cell that fights infection.
11. The process of adding a polyethylene glycol molecule to another molecule.
12. Hormone-like peptide, released by activated lymphocytes, that mediates immune response.
16. The generic name for Neupogen. Its mode of action increases production of neutrophils.
17. Interferon ___ enhances the oxidative metabolism of macrophages.
18. This technology process uses mice to mass-produce monoclonal antibodies.
22. The commonly used abbreviation for granulocyte macrophage colony stimulating factor.

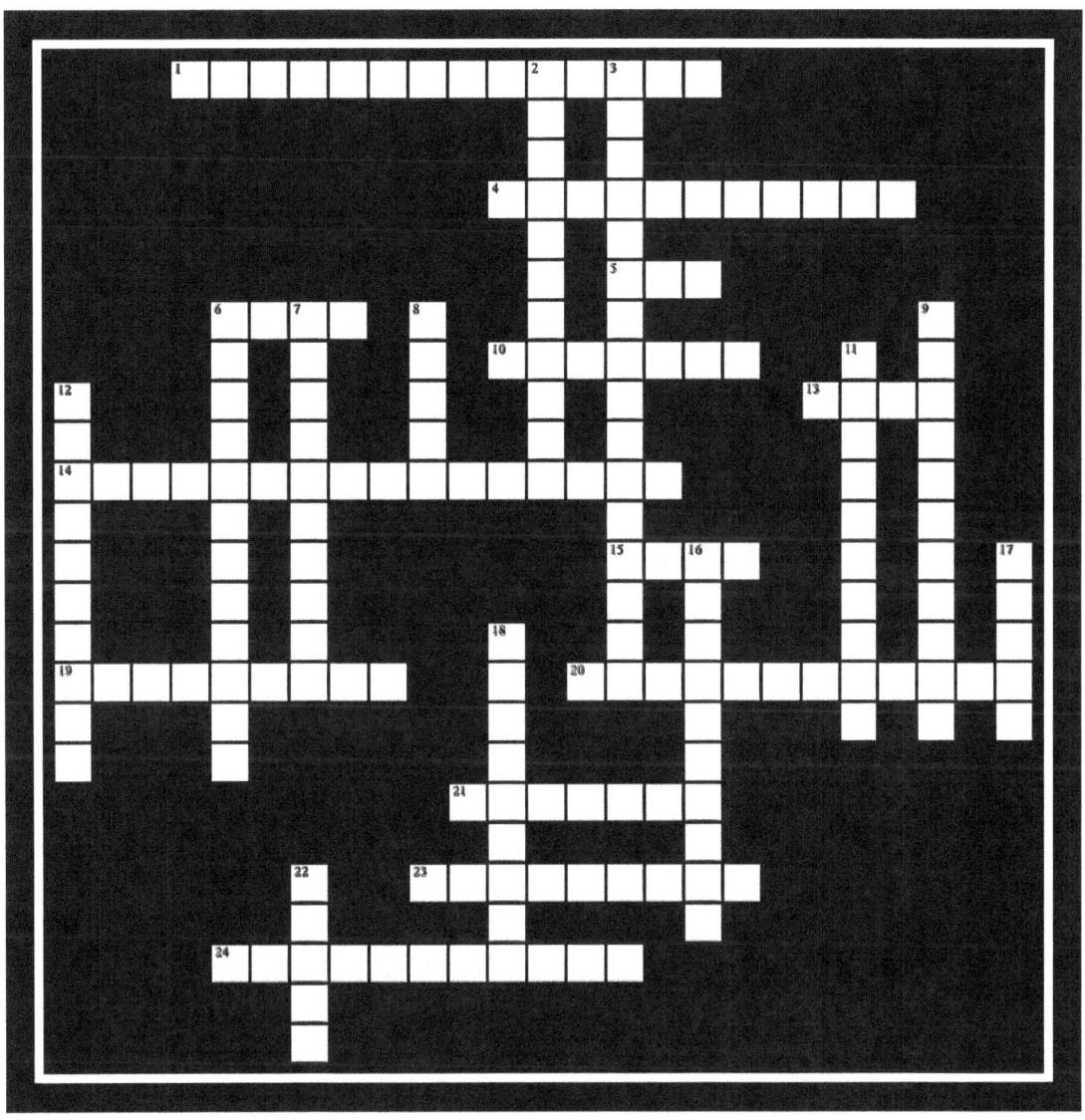

Pharmacology
Crossword Challenge
Antineoplastic Agents
Immune System Enhancers
Section X

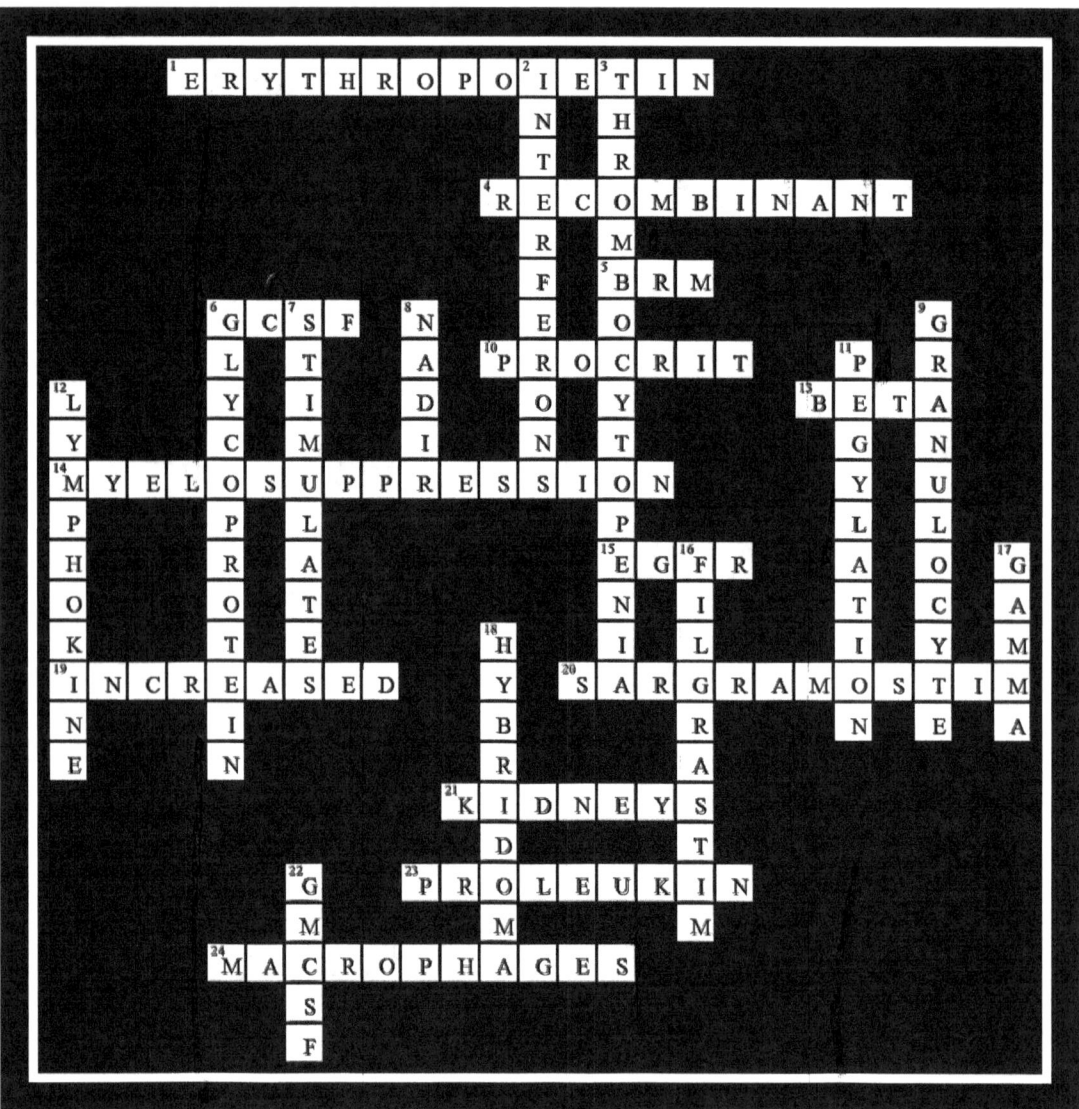

Pharmacology
Crossword Challenge
Antineoplastic Agents
Immune System Enhancers
Section X
Notes

Across

2. Benadryl's mode of action is to ___ histamine.
5. Commonly used abbreviation for this inhibitor, monoamine oxidase
8. These agents assist in shrinking nasal mucous membranes and reduce fluid secretion.
9. Commonly used drug for relief of allergic rhinitis and urticaria.
11. An inflammation of the mucous membranes of one or more of the maxillary, frontal, ethmoid or sphenoid sinuses.
13. These drugs loosen bronchial secretions so they can be eliminated by coughing.
14. Allergic rhinitis is often referred to as this type of fever.
15. A commonly used drug for rhinitis, generic name of triprolidine/pseudoephedrine.
18. A narcotic antitussive. The generic name for Hycodan.
22. A non-narcotic antitussive that suppresses the cough center. It does not depress respiration.
23. These drugs act on the cough-control center in the medulla to suppress the cough reflex.
24. Pseudoephedrine may ___ the effect of beta blockers.
25. A trade name for diphenhydramine, commonly used antihistamine.

Down

1. The generic name for Robitussin. Loosens bronchial secretions.
2. The generic term for Rhinocort, an intranasal glucocorticoid with anti-inflammatory action.
3. This generation of antihistamines are frequently called nonsedating antihistamines.
4. The generic name for Beconase. Used to treat allergic rhinitis.
6. This is the phase in which oxygen passes through the airways.
7. Drugs having an action antagonistic to that of histamine on either H1 or H2 receptors
10. This part of the respiratory tract consists of the nares, nasal cavity, pharynx and larynx.
12. The common cold is the most prevalent type of ___.
16. Trade name for cetirizine.
17. A drug capable of combining with receptors to initiate drug actions; it possesses affinity and intrinsic activity.
19. A term used to describe watery nasal discharge.
20. A term used to describe hives.
21. Lung compliance is the lung volume based on the unit of pressure in the ___.

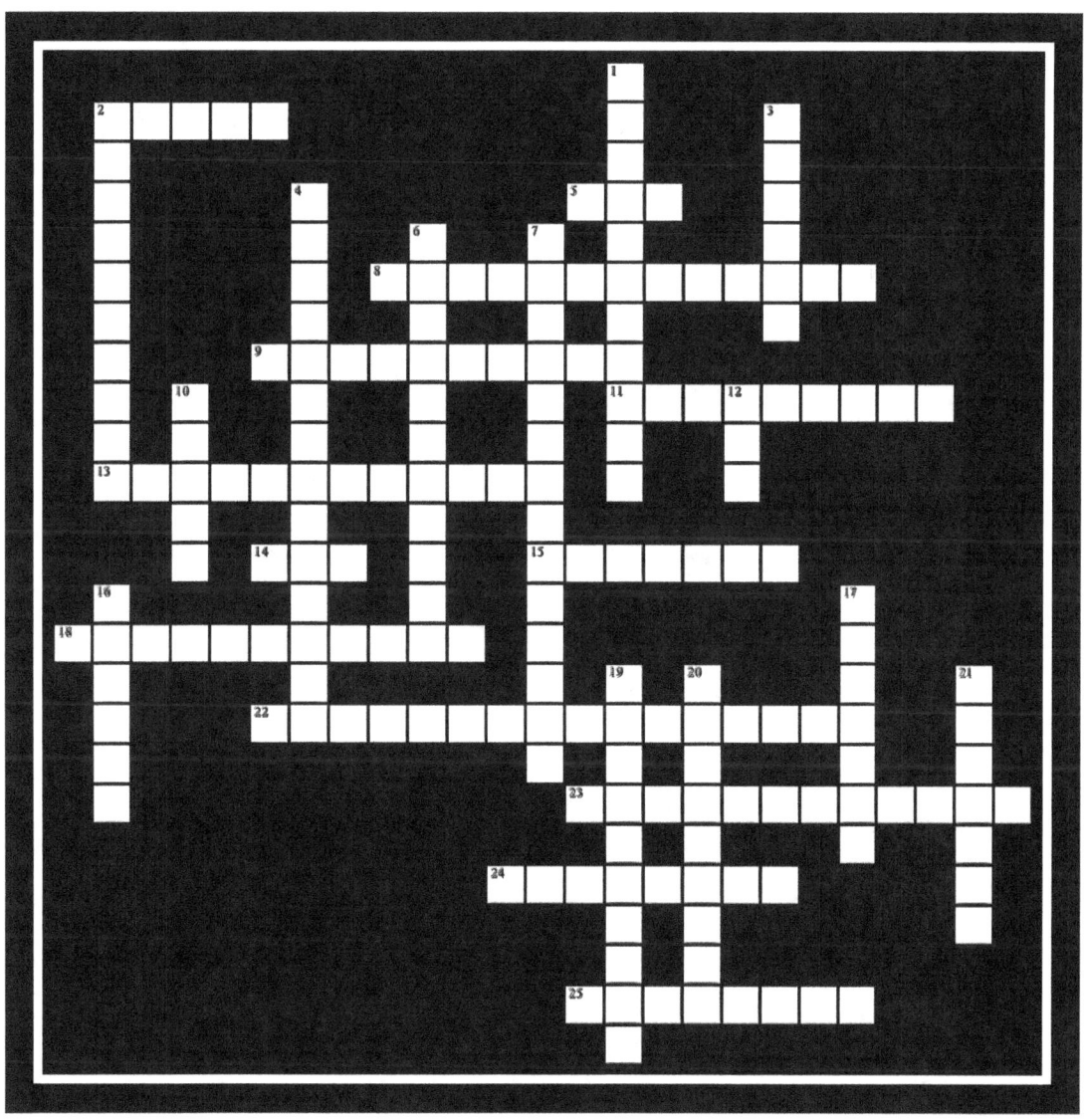

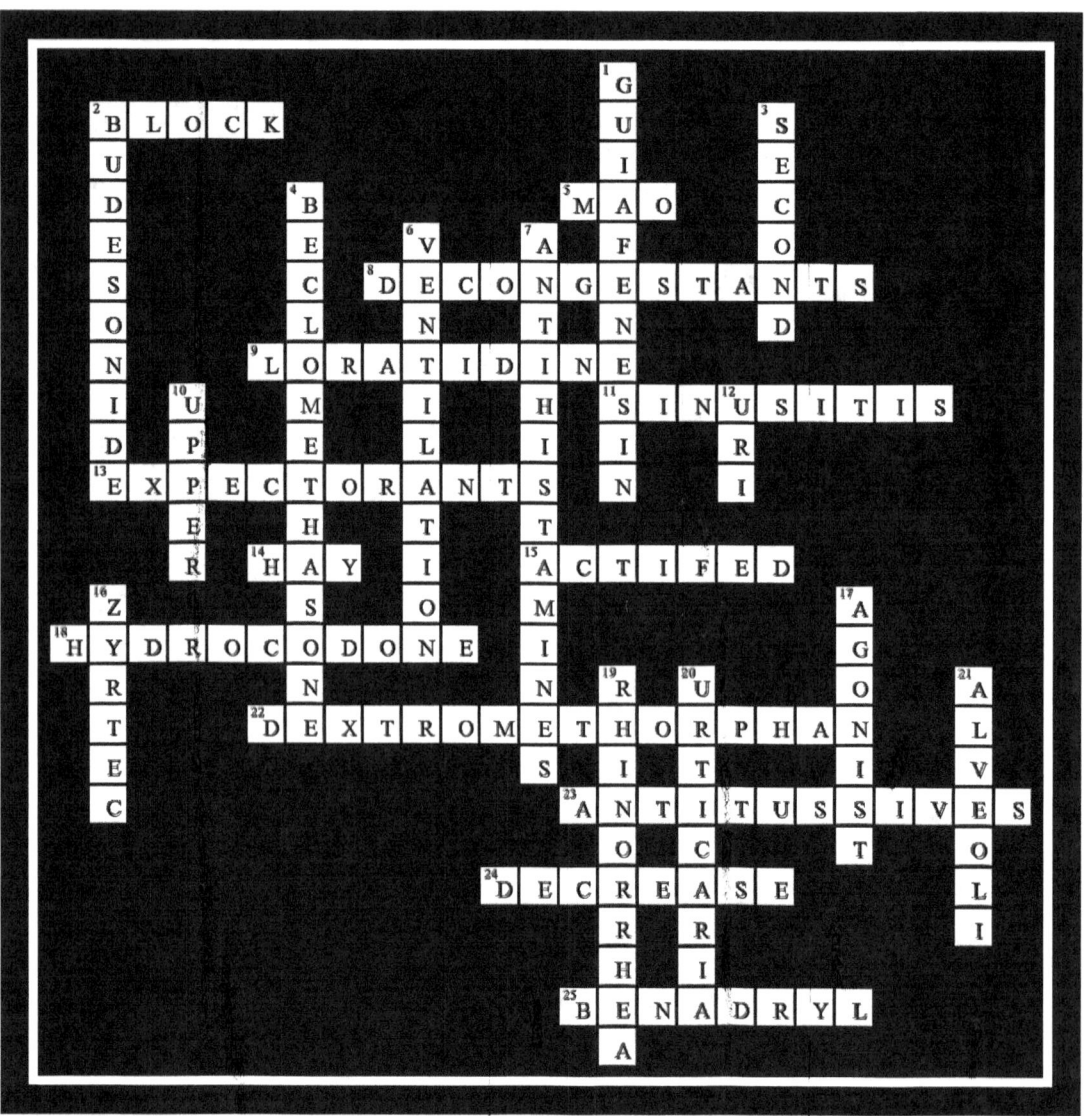

Pharmacology
Crossword Challenge
Respiratory Agents
Upper Respiratory Disorders
Section XI
Notes

Pharmacology
Crossword Challenge
Respiratory Agents
Lower Respiratory Disorders
Section XI

Across

3. These agents cause an increase in the diameter of the bronchus or bronchial tubes.

5. This herb may increase the effect of theophylline and may cause toxicity.

8. This is the generic term for Singulair, a bronchodilator which inhibits smooth muscle contraction.

10. A condition of the lung characterized by increase beyond the normal in the size of air spaces distal to the terminal bronchiole.

11. This drug relaxes the smooth muscles of the bronchi, used for bronchial asthma.

12. Abbreviation for cyclic adenosine monophosphate.

14. Isuprel, a beta-adrenergic, may be confused with this drug which is a nitrate vasodilator.

16. This is a trade name for the combination of ipratropium with albuterol used to increase bronchodilation.

18. These members of the corticosteroid family are used to treat asthma.

21. An inflammatory disorder of the airway walls associated with a varying amount of airway obstruction.

23. An abnormal dilation of the bronchi and bronchioles.

24. This drug acts by inhibiting the release of histamine to prevent an asthma reaction. The generic name for Intal.

Down

1. This drug is an enzyme that digests DNA in thick sputum secretions of patients with cystic fibrosis (2 words).

2. Commonly used abbreviation for chronic obstructive pulmonary disease.

4. These act like detergents to liquefy/loosen thick mucous so it may be expectorated.

6. These are used when infection develops from retained mucous secretions.

7. The best medication for a patient with an acute bronchospasm.

9. The generic term for Alupent. Its mode of action is to relax smooth muscle of bronchi.

13. Metaproterenol is well absorbed in the ___ tract.

15. Isoproterenol is administered by this route.

17. This type of asthma is a COPD characterized by period of bronchospasm with wheezing.

19. The generic term for Xopenex used in the treatment of acute bronchospasm.

20. Sympathomimetics increase cAMP, causing ___ of the bronchioles.

22. Cromolyn and nedocromil are drugs used to treat asthma in ___.

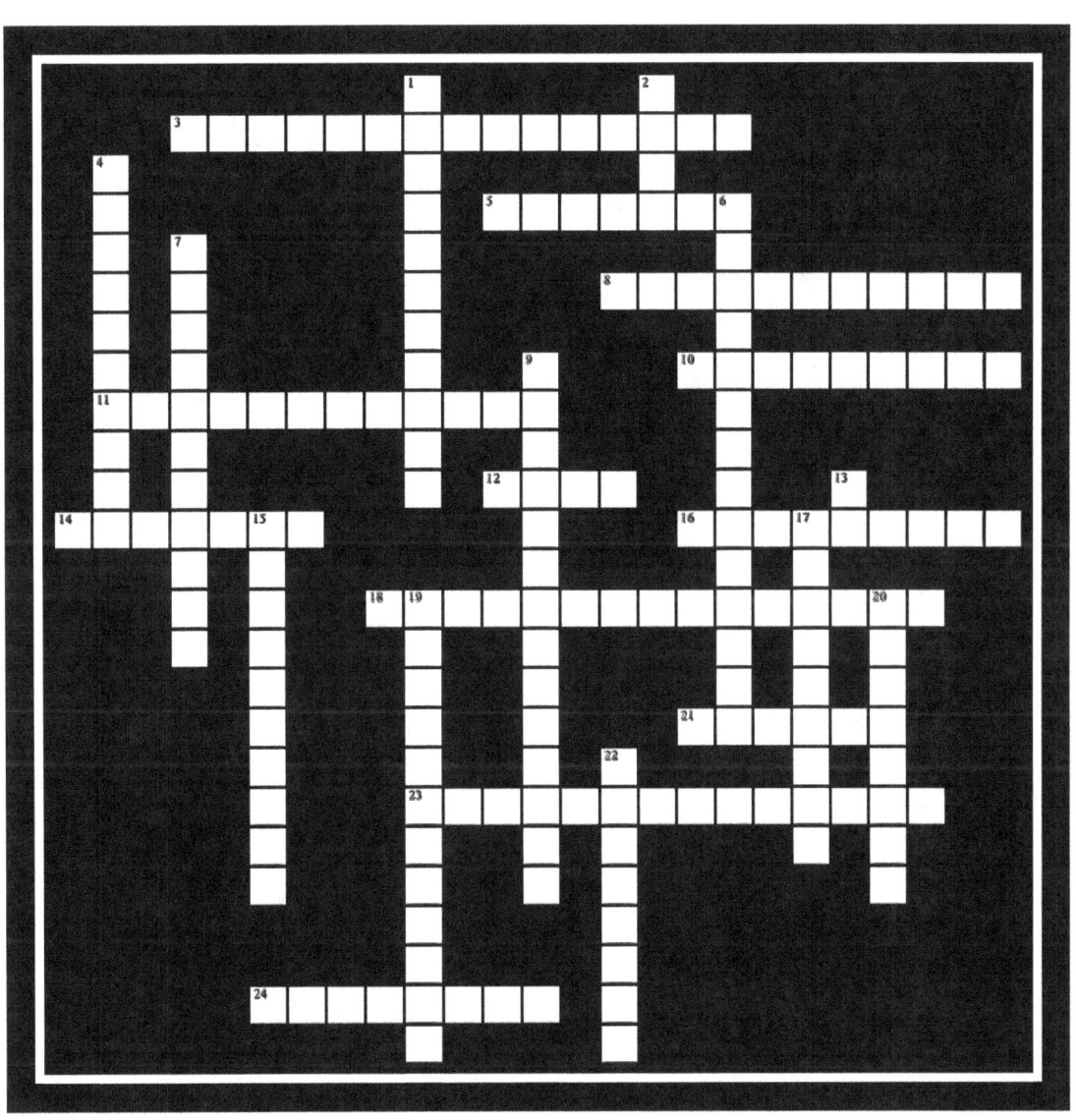

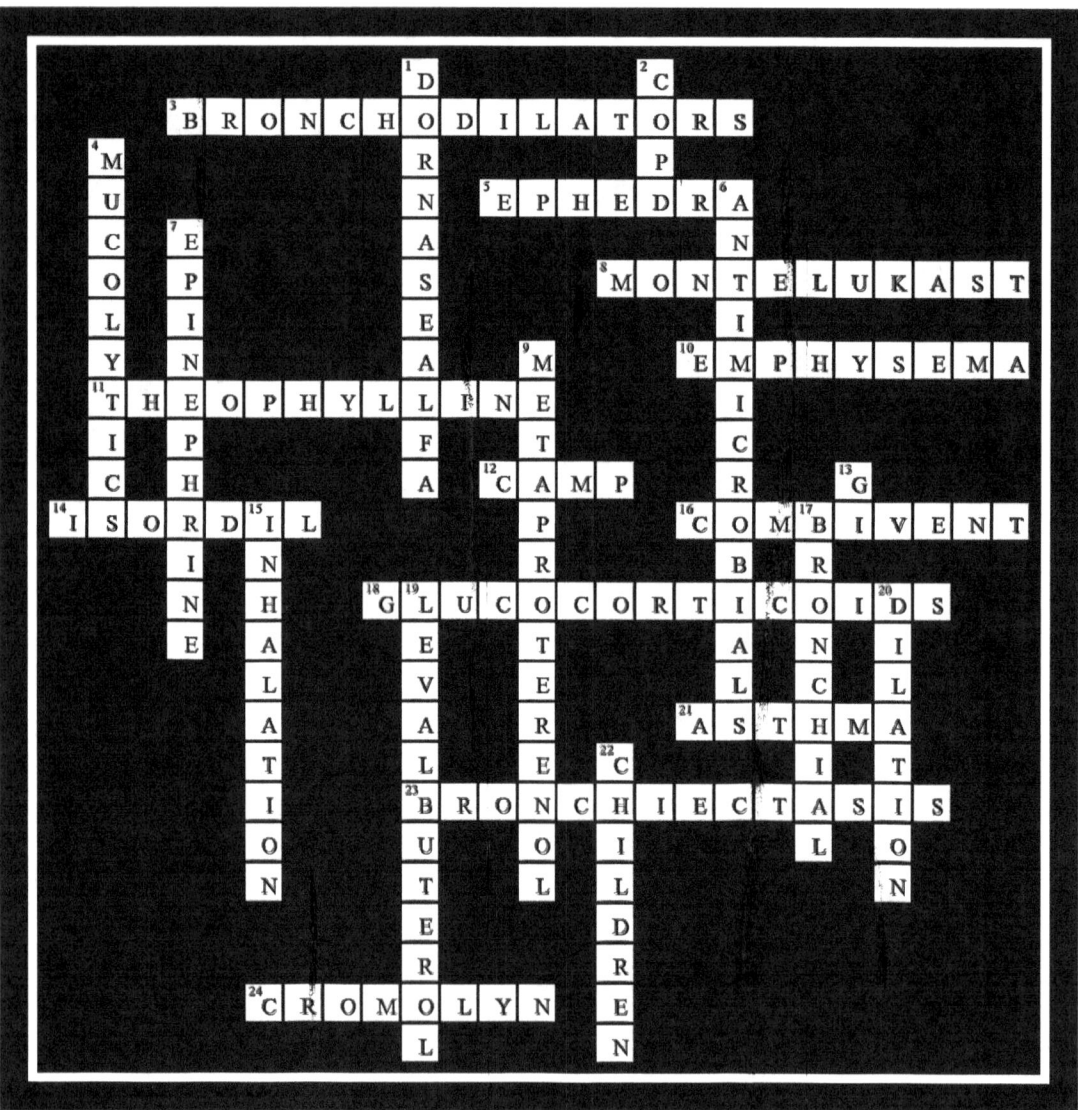

Pharmacology
Crossword Challenge
Respiratory Agents
Lower Respiratory Disorders
Section XI
Notes

Across

5. This type of angina occurs during rest.

9. A term used to describe a low serum potassium level.

10. Verapamil belongs to this class of channel blockers.

12. This negative action decreases conduction of the heart cells.

14. A common symptom that often occurs with taking a nitrate.

15. The term used to describe myocardial contraction.

18. Any deviation from the normal rate or pattern of the heartbeat.

19. This positive action increases myocardial contraction stroke volume.

21. These drugs are used to treat angina pectoris.

22. Beta blockers are effective as antianginals because they cause the heart rate to ___.

24. This drug is the antidote for digitalis toxicity.

25. The generic term for Bretylol. It prolongs repolarization.

Down

1. The term used to describe peripheral vascular resistance.

2. The generic term for Norvasc, a calcium channel blocker.

3. The generic term for Inderal.

4. This glycoside is contraindicated in the case of ventricular dysrhythmia. It is used to treat heart failure, atrial tachycardia.

6. Generic term for Betapace, a beta-adrenergic blocker used for ventricular dysrhythmias.

7. This group of drugs is used to correct atrial fibrillation/flutter. They inhibit the sodium-potassium pump.

8. The return of cell membrane potential to resting after depolarization.

11. This is the term for heart muscle.

13. This negative action decreases heart rate.

16. The term used to describe rapid heart beat.

17. Generic term for Cardizem, a calcium channel blocker used for PSVT, atrial flutter/fibrillation.

20. These antianginals cause generalized vascular and coronary vasodilation.

23. Lidocaine belongs to this class of channel blocker.

Pharmacology
Crossword Challenge
Cardiovascular Agents
Glycosides, Antianginals & Antidysrhythmics
Section XII

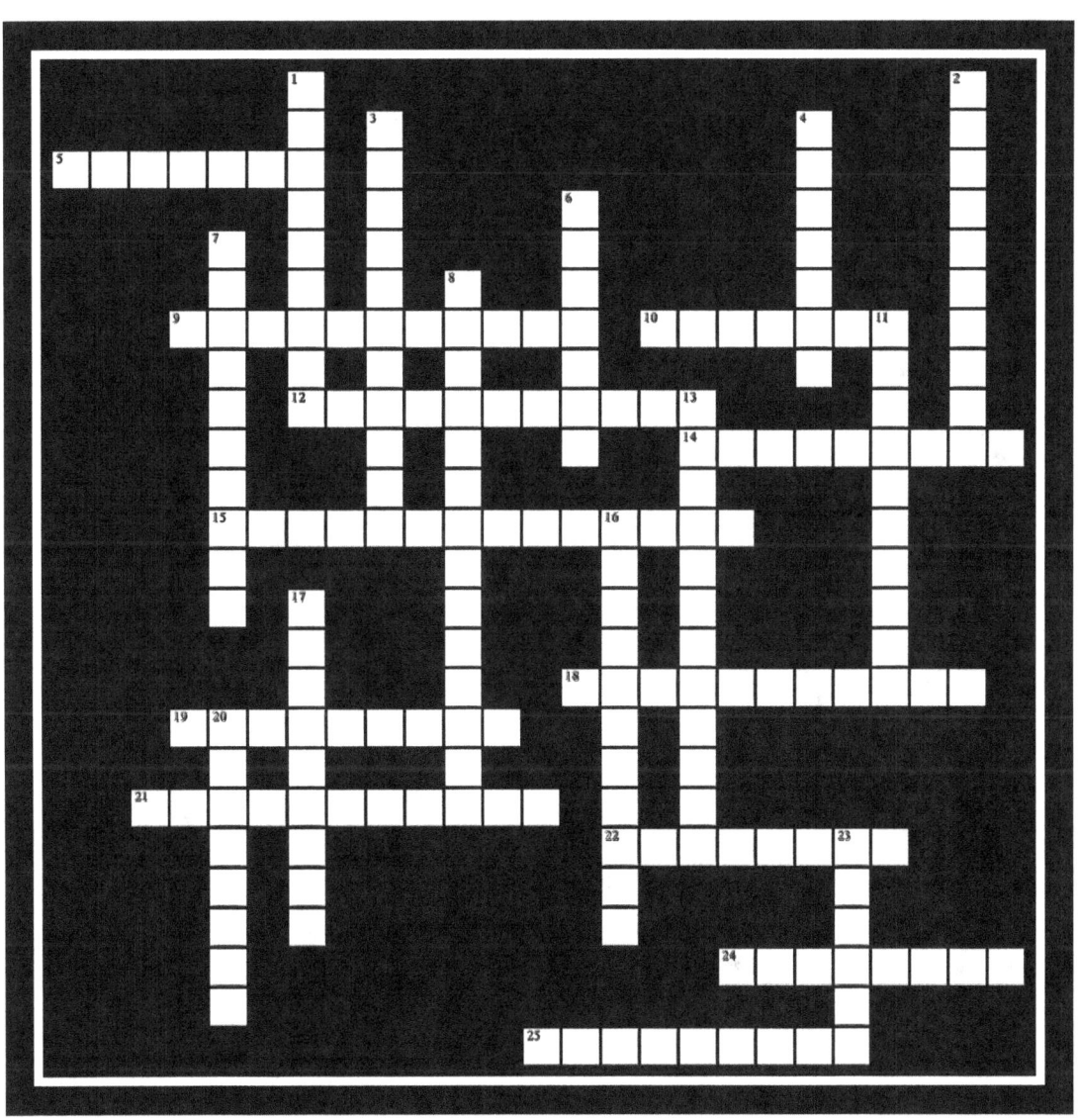

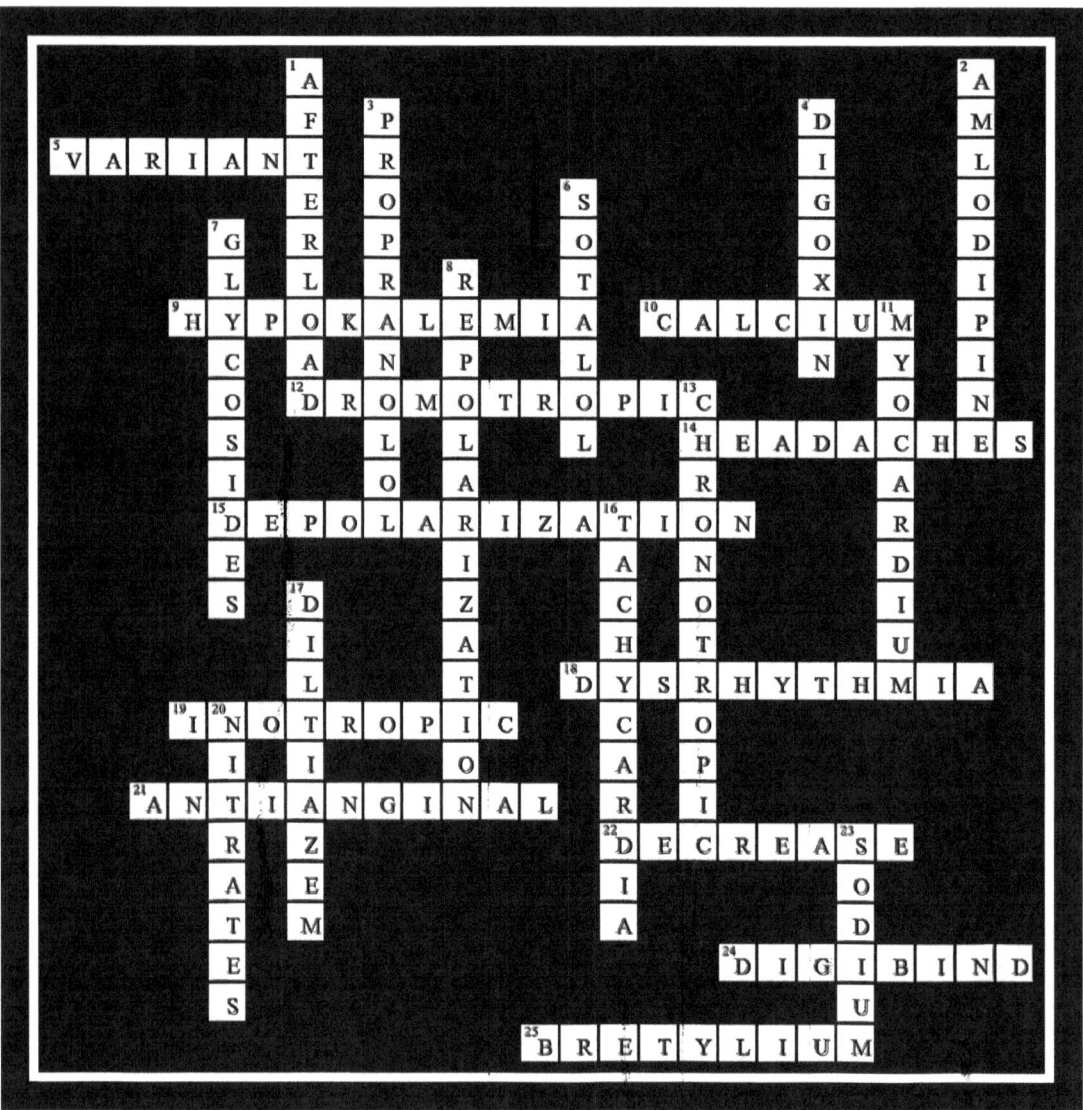

Pharmacology
Crossword Challenge
Cardiovascular Agents
Glycosides, Antianginals & Antidysrhythmics
Section XII
Notes

Across

3. Commonly used abbreviation for hydrochlorothiazide.

5. The net movement of a solvent, which is water in living systems, through a selectively permeable membrane.

6. The generic term for Lozol, a long-acting thiazide and may be classified as a loop diuretic.

8. This is the double-walled epithelial cup also called the glomerular capsule.

9. The diuretics that promote potassium retention are called potassium ___ diuretics.

10. Thiazides affect the ___ tubule.

12. This condition may occur with patients taking 50 mg of hydrochlorothiazide and digoxin 0.25 daily.

13. The generic term for Bumex, a high-ceiling, loop, diuretic.

14. The term used to describe marked decrease in urine output.

17. The generic term for Aldactone, a potassium-sparing diuretic.

20. A name given to the nephron loop which extends into the medulla, then loops up to the cortex.

21. Generic term for Diamox, carbonic anhydrase inhibitor, used to treat edema.

22. Diuretics have this effect because they promote sodium and water loss.

23. This osmotic is used for oliguria and to prevent acute renal failure.

Down

1. Osmotic, mercurial and CAI diuretics affect the ___ tubule.

2. This short-acting thiazide is used for peripheral edema. Its trade name is Diuril.

4. Maxzide is a combinatioin of hydrochlorothiazide and ___.

7. This term is used to describe sodium loss in the urine.

9. This term is used to describe loss of sodium and chloride.

11. A term used to describe elevated serum uric acid level.

14. The concentration of a solution expressed in osmoles of solute particles per kilogram of soluent.

15. Triamterene and hydrochlorothiazide may be prescribed to cause the serum potassium level to ___.

16. Potassium-sparing diuretics act on the ___ tubules.

18. The diuretics that promote potassium excretion are classified as potassium ___ diuretics.

19. A term used to describe increased urine flow.

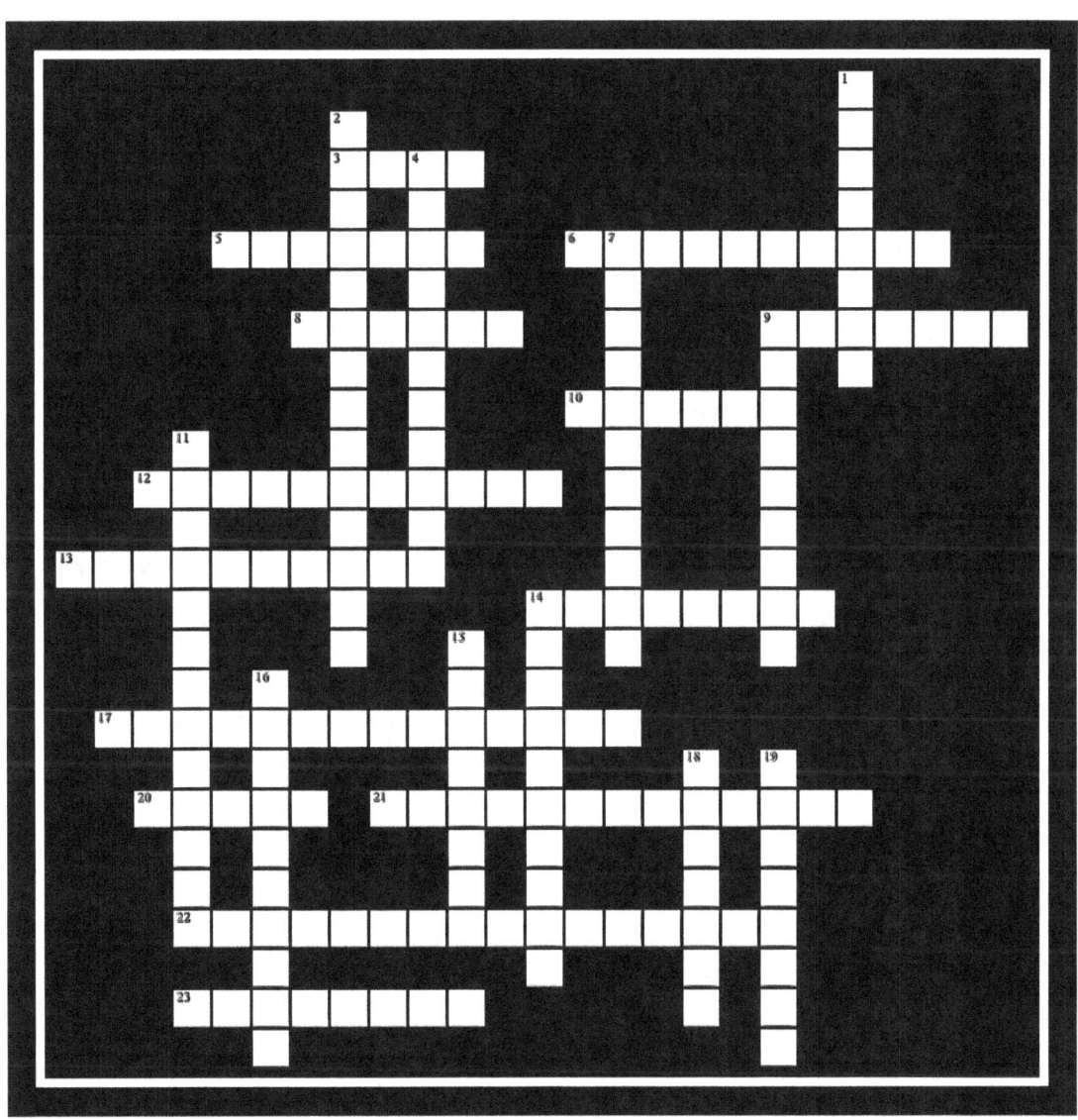

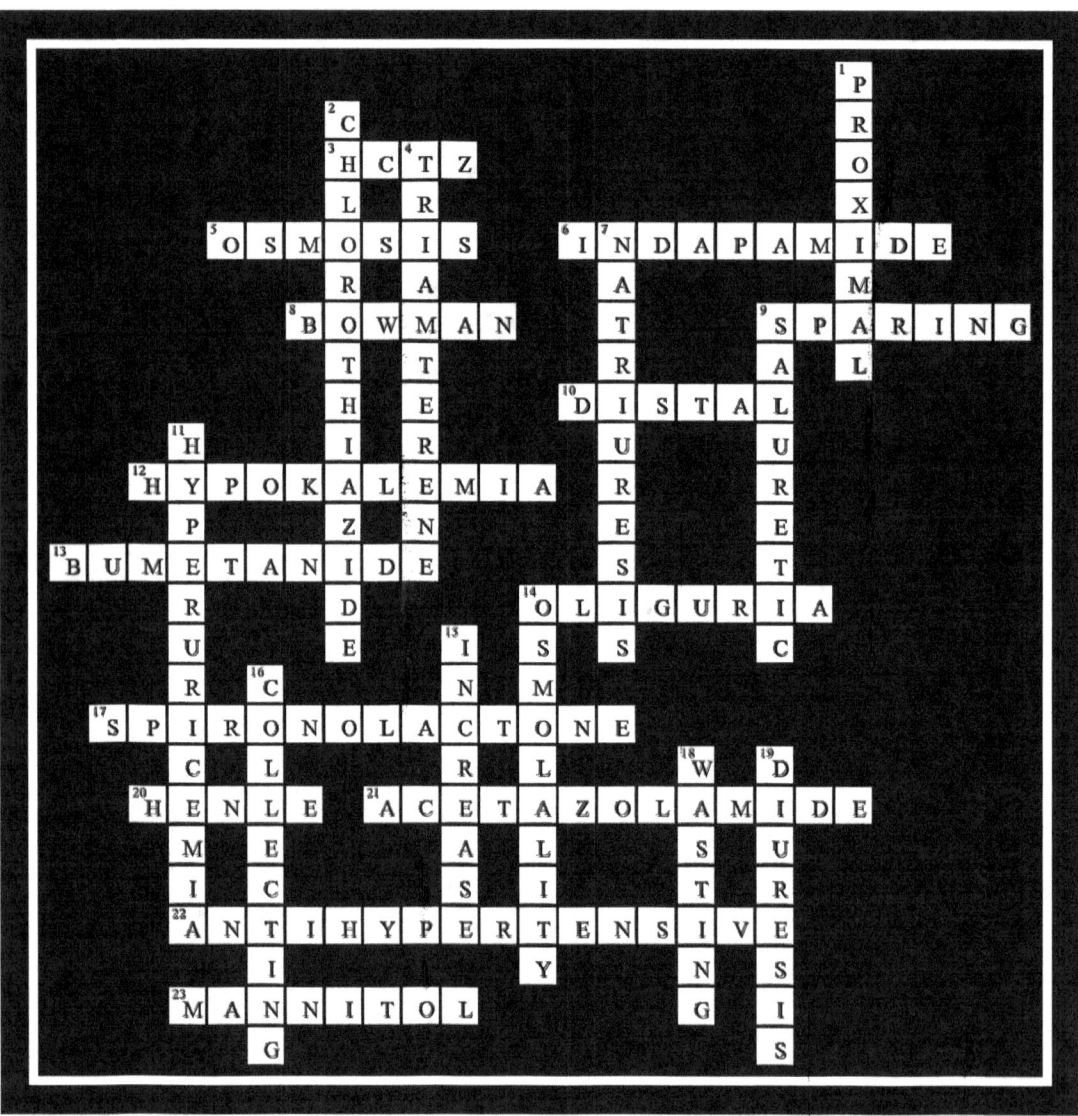

Pharmacology
Crossword Challenge
Cardiovascular Agents
Diuretics
Section XII
Notes

Across

6. Commonly used abbreviation for hypertension.
7. This drug, an antihypertensive, may be easily confused with Dioval, an estrogen hormone.
8. Trade name of Tekturna. It binds with renin, causes reduction of angiotensin I and II.
10. Ten percent of hypertension cases are related to renal & endocrine disorders and are classified as ___ hypertension.
14. This herb antagonizes the effects of antihypertensive drugs.
15. The generic name for Monopril. Reduces peripheral resistance and improves cardiac output.
16. Commonly used abbreviation for angiotensin-converting enzyme.
18. The generic name for Cozaar. It is a potent vasodilator and inhibits the binding of angiotensin II.
20. The generic name for Minipress. Its mode of action is to dilate peripheral blood vessels via blocking alpha-adrenergic receptors.
21. Centrally acting alpha2 agonists cause the sympathetic response to ___ from the brainstem to the peripheral vessels.
24. The generic name for Inderal. It is a nonselective beta1 and beta2.
25. The generic name for Coreg. It is an alpha-blocker; nonselective beta1 and beta2.

Down

1. Denoting antagonism to or inhibition of adrenergic nerve activity.
2. The generic name for Aldomet. Used for stage 1 to 3 hypertension. Long acting. May be used alone or in combination.
3. Alcohol increases these secretions causing the production of angiotension II.
4. The most frequent diuretic that is combined with an antihypertensive drug.
5. Generic name for Atacand. May be used for patients who do not respond to ACE inhibitors.
9. The generic name for Lopressor. Its mode of action is to promote blood pressure reduction via beta-blocking effect.
11. The generic name for Procardia. For HTN & angina pectoris, a potent calcium channel blocker.
12. Selective alpha-adrenergic blockers cause this to happen to arterioles and venules.
13. Weight loss and a restriction of this in a patient's diet may result in decreased hypertension.
17. The generic name for Vasotec. Used in hypertensive emergencies.
19. The term used to describe reduced peripheral resistance.
22. A common side effect of ACE inhibitors is a ___.
23. Commonly used abbreviation for very low-density lipoproteins.

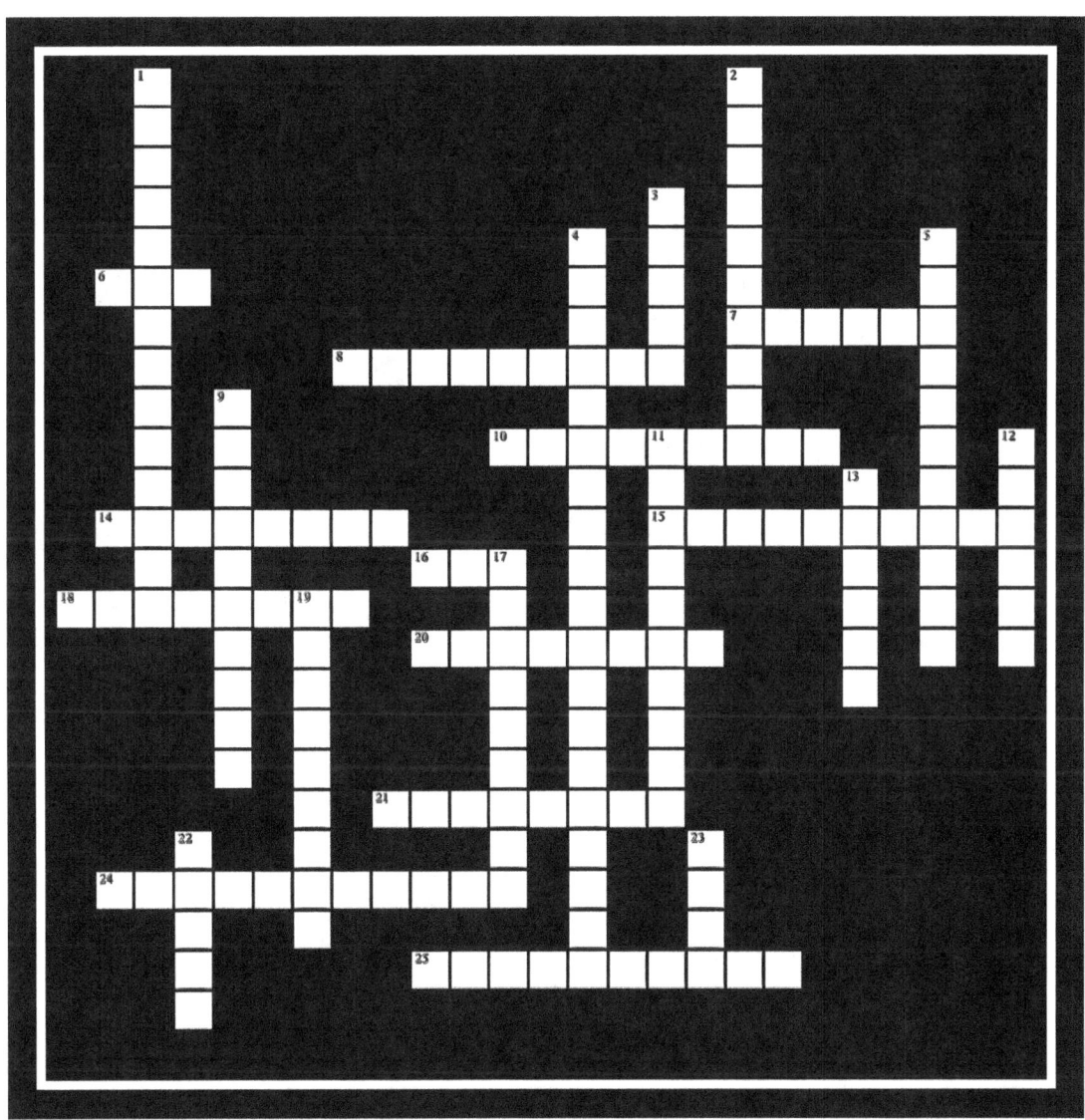

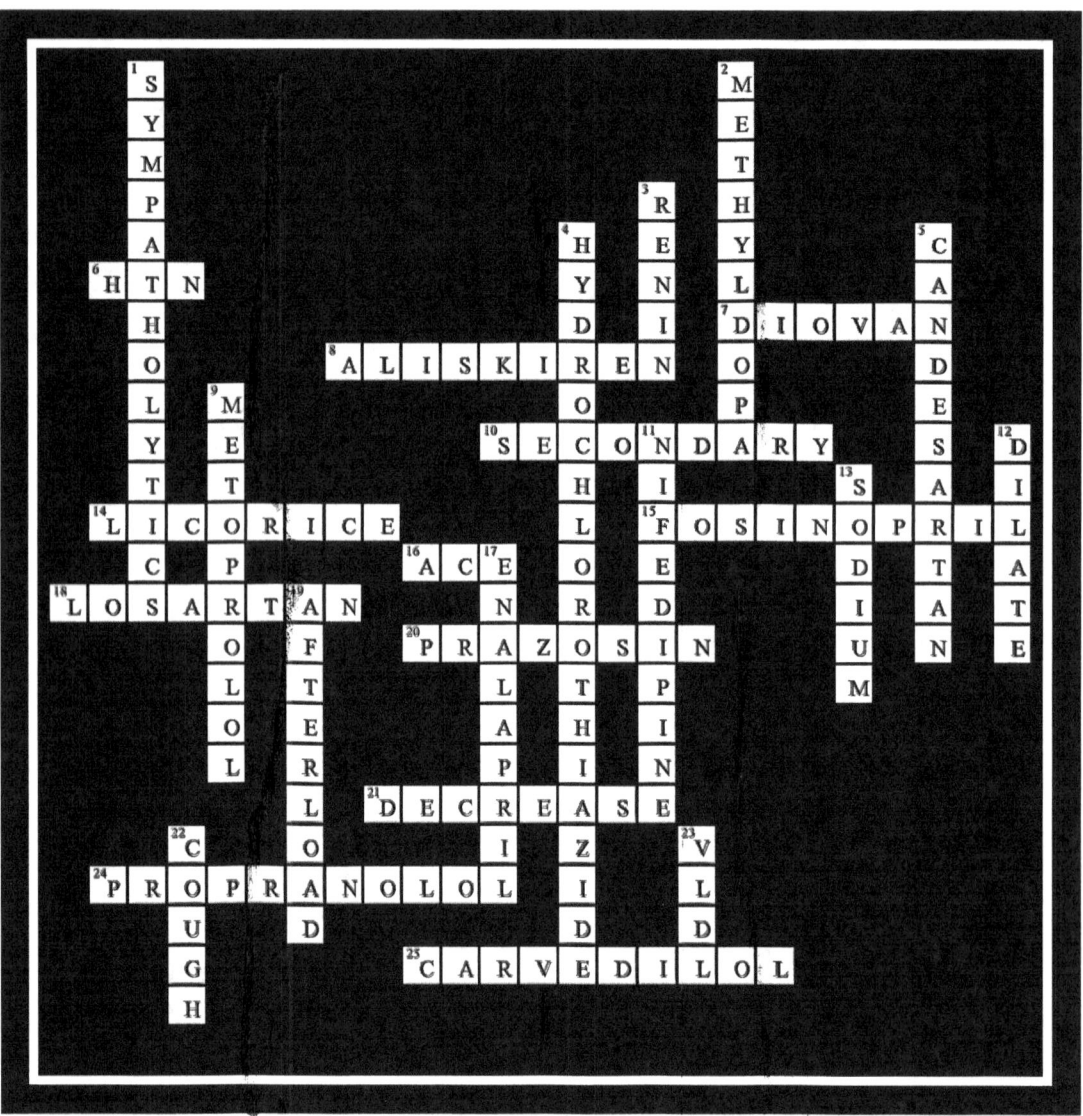

Pharmacology
Crossword Challenge
Cardiovascular Agents
Antihypertensives
Section XII
Notes

Pharmacology
Crossword Challenge
Cardiovascular Agents
Anticoagulants, Antiplatelets, Thrombolytics
Section XII

Across

2. LMWH route of administration.

5. The generic name for Coumadin.

8. This drug should be used instead of aspirin for patients taking warfarin.

10. Commonly used abbreviation for deep venous thrombosis.

13. Anaphylaxis occurs more frequently with this agent than with other thrombolytics.

14. This is the major adverse effect of warfarin.

15. Clumping together of platelets to form a clot.

17. An enzyme which digests the fibrin matrix of clots.

18. An area of necrosis resulting from a sudden insufficiency of arterial or venous blood supply.

19. Formation of a clot in an arterial or venous vessel.

22. This group of drugs is used to prevent thrombosis in the arteries by suppressing platelet aggregation.

24. Trade name ReoPro, used primarily for preventing reocclusion of coronary arteries.

25. This herb may decrease the effects of warfarin, thereby decreasing the INR.

Down

1. Trade name of Plavix. An antiplatelet used for prevention of thromboembolism. It prevents ADP from binding with ADP platelet receptor.

3. Commonly used abbreviation for activated partial thromboplastin time, lab tests to detect deficiency in clotting.

4. This lab test measures the time it takes blood to clot.

6. This thrombolytic promotes conversion of plasminogen to plasmin.

7. An antidote for heparin.

9. Group of drugs used to inhibit clot formation.

11. The generic name for Lovenox, one of four LMWHs.

12. The term used to describe fibrin breakdown.

16. This group of drugs convert plasminogen to plasmin which destroys the fibrin in the blood clot.

20. Warfarin's route of administration.

21. A natural substance in the liver that prevents clot formation.

23. The commonly used abbreviation for tissue plasminogen activator.

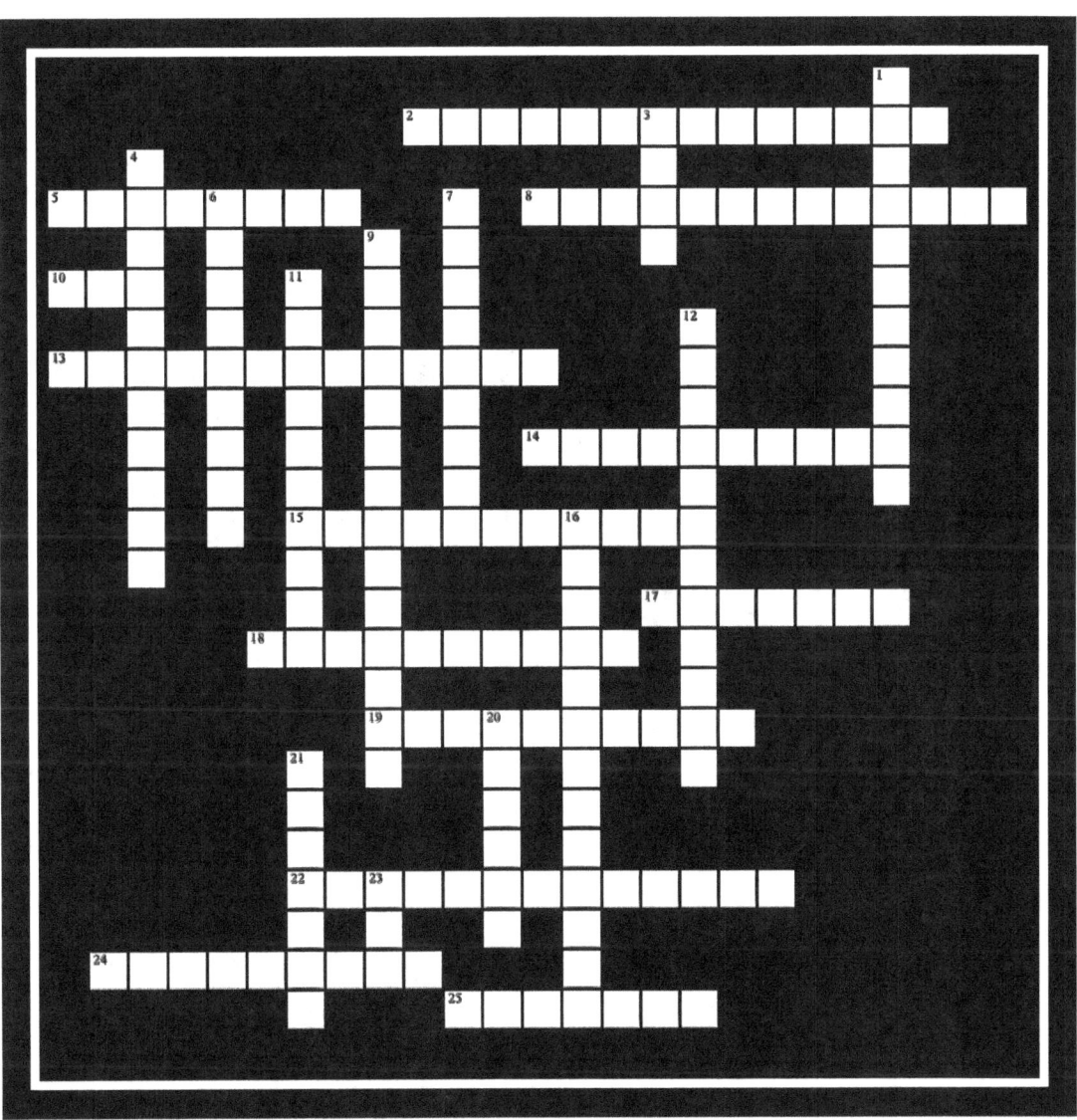

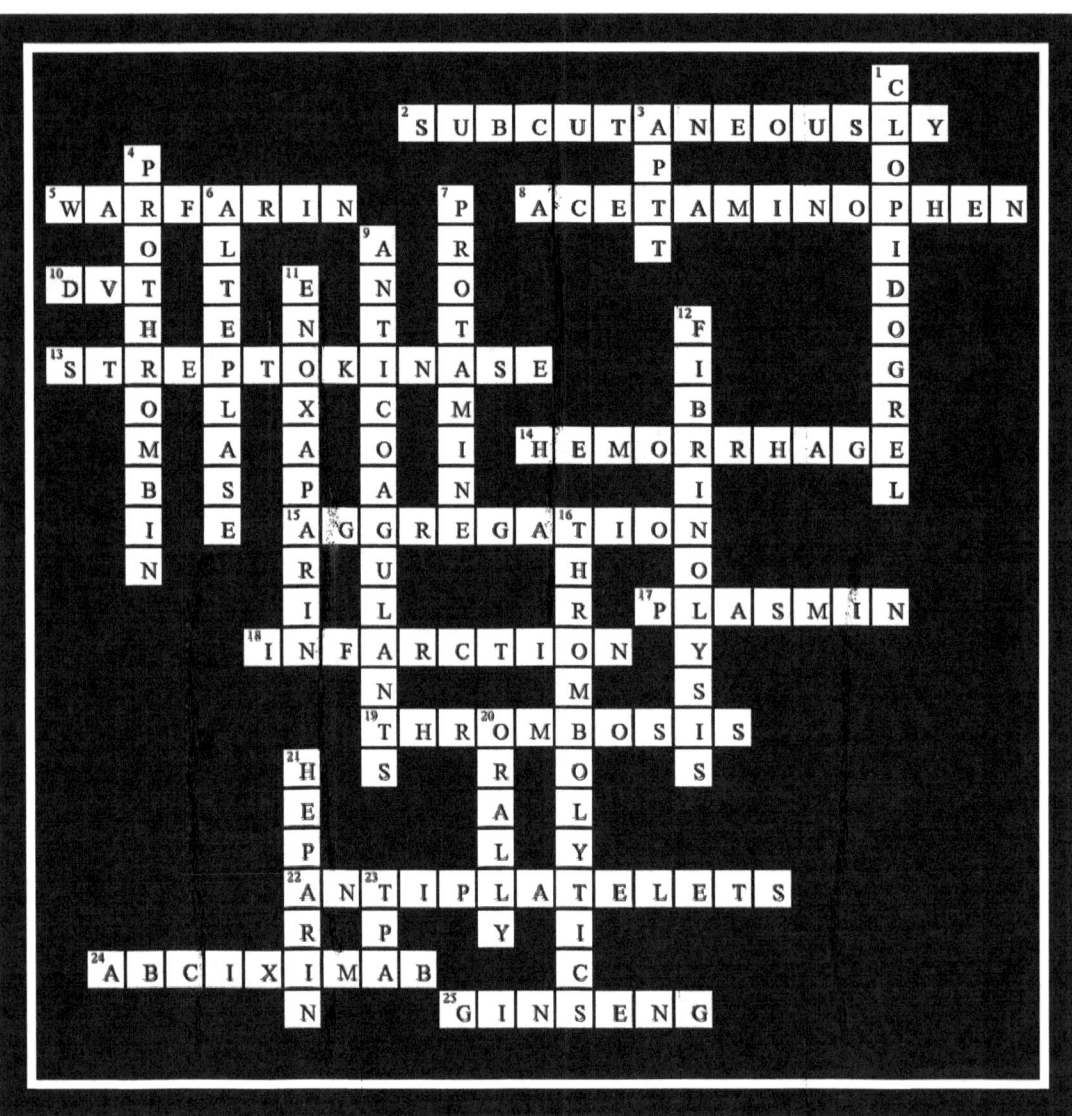

Pharmacology
Crossword Challenge
Cardiovascular Agents
Anticoagulants, Antiplatelets, Thrombolytics
Section XII
Notes

Across

1. A total intake of this in your diet should be limited to 30% or less of caloric intake.

6. The generic name for Tricor, used in treatment of type IV and V hyperlipidemia.

8. Another term for fibric acid.

9. This group of drugs inhibits cholesterol synthesis in the liver and slightly decreases the concentration of HDL.

11. The generic name for Lipitor. Its mode of action is to inhibit HMG-CoA reductase.

12. This term describes cholesterol, triglycerides and phospholipids.

15. These are large lipid droplets of reprocessed lipid synthesized and contain triacylglycerols.

16. Pentoxifylline (Trental) falls under the classification of this agent.

18. An excess of one or more lipids in the blood.

19. The commonly used abbreviation for very low-density lipoprotein.

20. A trade name for nicotinic acid where doses are 100 times higher than RDA to lower VLDL.

22. This adverse reaction may occur in patients taking statins.

Down

1. The generic name for Lescol, belongs to the group of statins.

2. The generic name for Priscoline. Used for neonatal pulmonary hypertension.

3. The generic name for Lopid, a bile-acid sequestrant.

4. The primary cause of peripheral arterial/vascular disease.

5. The generic name for Crestor. Antilipidemic which may cut LDL in half.

7. Elevated levels of this have been associated with certain forms of heart disease.

10. Lipids are composed of cholesterol, phospholipids and ___.

13. This activity is an important aspect of nonpharmacologic method to reduce cholesterol.

14. This is a trade name for the combination of ezetimibe and simvastatin. Decreases absorption of cholesterol in the small intestine.

17. The generic name for Zetia, a cholesterol absorption inhibitor.

21. This the abbreviation for the "friendly" lipoprotein.

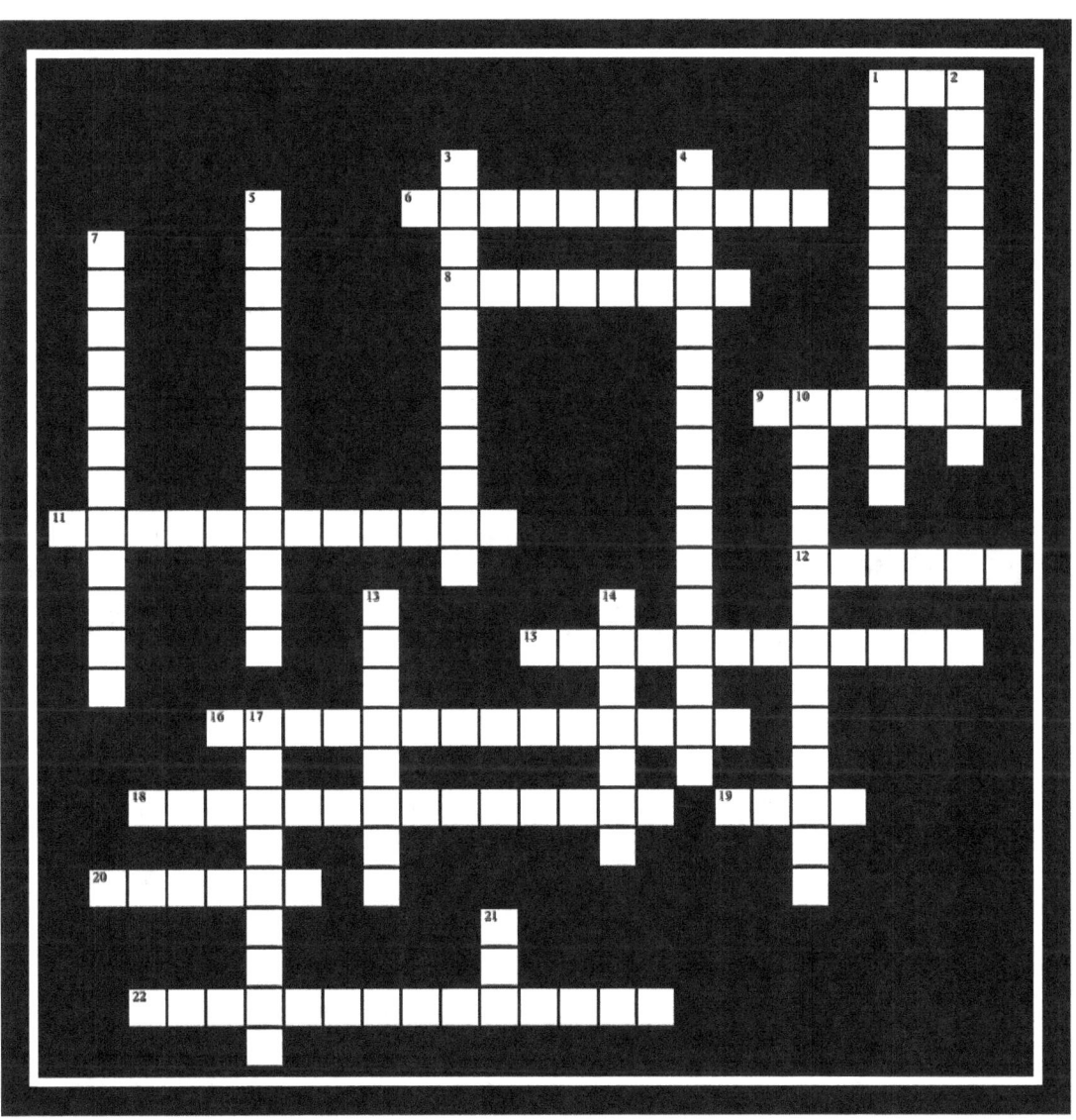

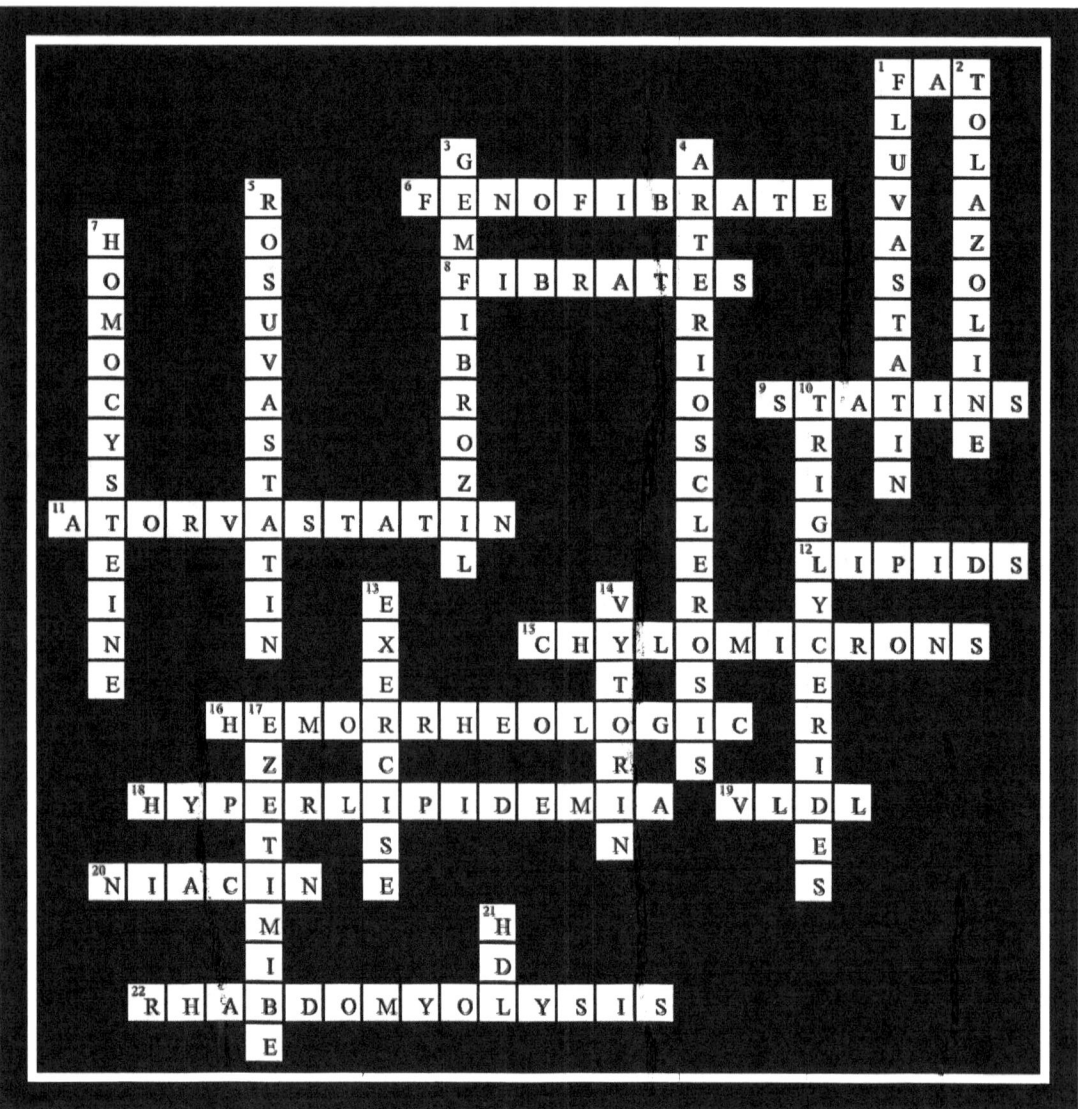

Pharmacology
Crossword Challenge
Cardiovascular Agents
Antilipidemics, Peripheral Vasodilators
Section XII
Notes

Across

1. The active ingredients in marijuana, a treatment to alleviate nausea.
6. This antiemetic is primarily used for prevention of nausea and vomiting during surgical procedures. (Inapsine).
7. This salt belongs to the class of osmotic saline stimulants, commonly known as Epsom.
9. This bulk-forming laxative (the generic name for Metamucil) acts by drawing water into the intestine.
10. A term used to describe lubricants and stool softeners used to prevent constipation.
12. This group of antidiarrheals is given for severe diarrhea resulting from metastatic carcinoid tumors.
14. The generic name for Dramamine, primarily used to prevent motion sickness.
17. This emollient comes in three forms: Calcium, potassium and sodium. Used as a stool softener.
18. The generic name for Ativan, usually administered with the antiemetic metoclopramide.
20. These agents act by coating the wall of the GI tract and adsorbing bacterial or toxins.
21. Commonly used abbreviation for chemoreceptor trigger zone.
23. The generic name for Dulcolax, a stimulant, increases peristalsis by direct effect on smooth muscle of the intestine.
24. These agents are used to eliminate fecal matter.
25. The generic term for Antivert, is used to prevent nausea, vomiting and dizziness.

Down

2. When metoclopramide (Reglan) is given for nausea, the client is cautioned to avoid this.
3. The generic name for Lomotil, combined with atropine, its mode of action is to inhibit gastric motility.
4. An accumulation of hard fecal material in the large intestine.
5. This antiemetic, the generic name for Phenergan, blocks H1 receptor sites & inhibits chemoreceptor trigger zone.
8. A term used to describe vomiting.
11. These agents treat diarrhea and decrease hypermotility.
13. These agents decrease intestinal motility and decrease peristalsis.
15. This syrup induces vomiting after poisoning.
16. A commonly used evacuant given in preparation for GI examination.
19. Another term for antivomiting agents.
22. This adsorbent is given in the prevention of traveler's diarrhea.

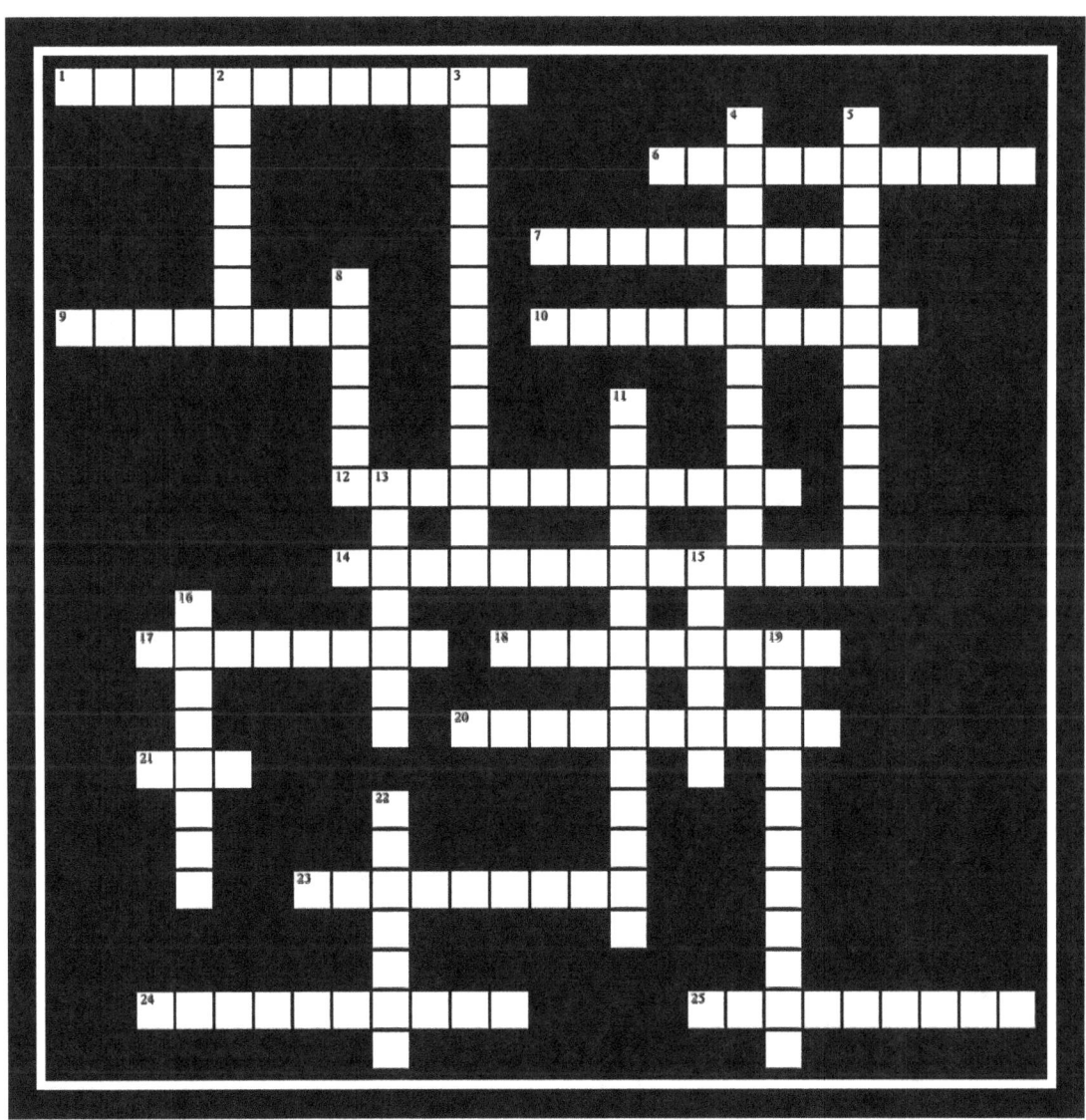

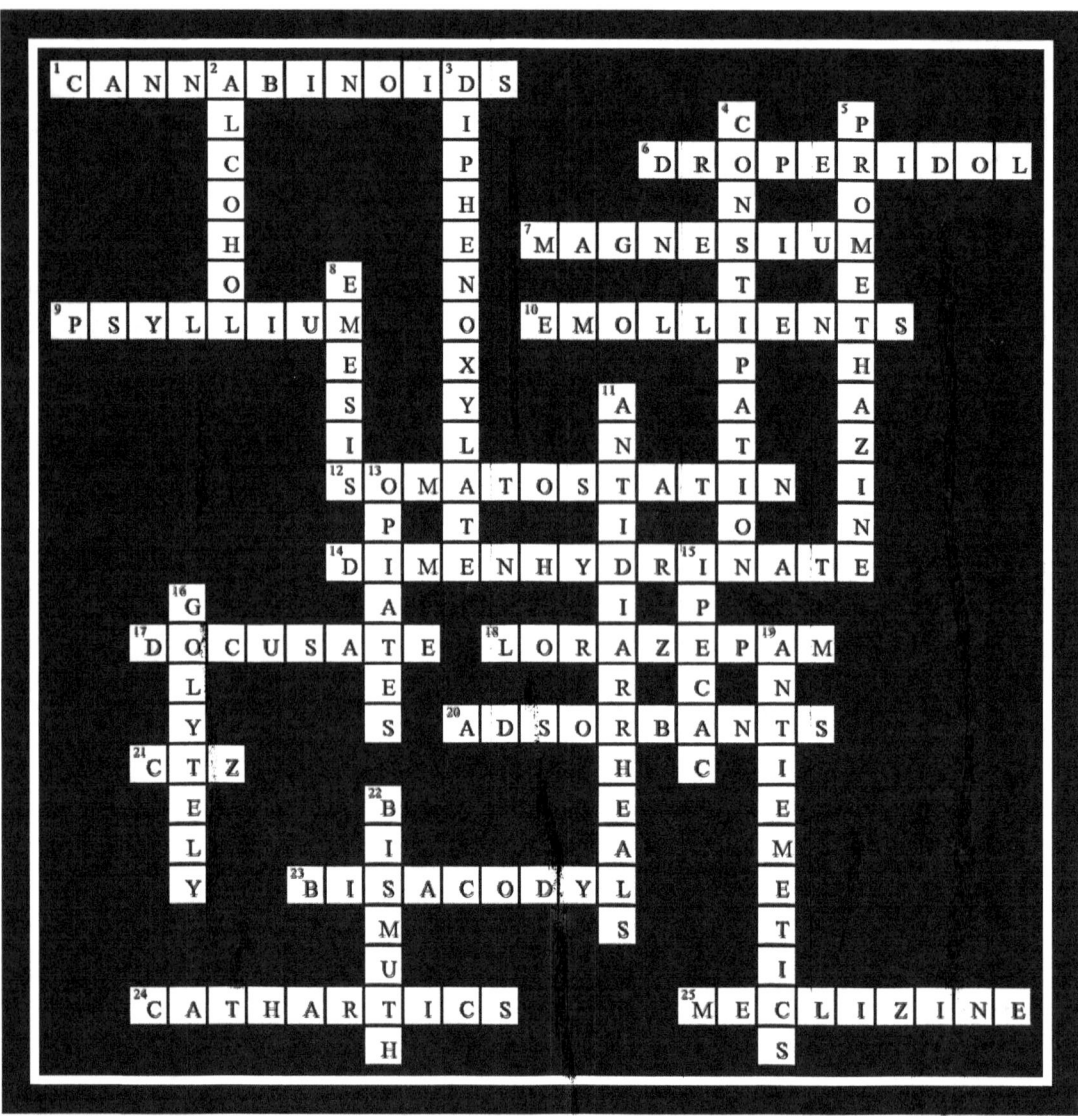

Pharmacology
Crossword Challenge
Gastrointestinal Agents
GI Tract Disorders
Section XIII
Notes

Pharmacology
Crossword Challenge
Gastrointestinal Agents
Antiulcer Drugs
Section XIII

Across

6. St. John's wort, when taken with tetracycline, may cause the risk of photosensitivity to ___ .
8. The generic name for Cytotec, a prostaglandin analogue.
9. The generic name for Flagyl. Used to treat H. pylori.
10. These agents are the treatment of choice for H. pylori.
14. A trade name for magnesium trisilicate, an antacid to relieve gastric disorders caused by hyperacidity.
16. This agent is a combination of clidinium bromide and chlordiazepoxide, used to decrease anxiety and GI distress.
17. The generic name for Prilosec. A proton pump inhibitor used to treat H. Pylori.
19. The generic name for Zantac, a histamine blocker which inhibits gastric acid secretion.
22. A commonly used abbreviation for gastric mucosal barrier.
23. This type of ulcer usually follows a critical situation such as trauma or major surgery.
24. This may be a side effect of taking famotidine.
25. The generic name for Tagamet, an H2 blocker, blocks about 70% of acid secretions for 4 hours.

Down

1. This carbonate antacid, with a trade name of Tums, is used to alleviate heartburn.
2. The generic name for Protonix, a proton pump inhibitor, used for treatment of gastric ulcers.
3. The generic name for Carafate, a pepsin inhibitor.
4. This type of ulcer is caused by hypersecretion of acid from the stomach passing into the duodenum.
5. The commonly used abbreviation for this disorder, an inflammation or erosion of the esophageal mucosa caused by reflux of the gastric mucosa.
7. This type of ulcer results from reflux of acidic gastric secretions into the esophagus.
11. This anticholinergic tincture is used to treat peptic ulcer.
12. This group of antiulcer drugs relieves pain by decreasing GI motility and secretions.
13. This group of antiulcer drugs reduces vagal stimulation and decreases anxiety.
15. These agents promote ulcer healing by neutralizing hydrochloric acid and reducing pepsin activity.
18. This type of ulcer is a broad term for an ulcer occurring in the esophagus, stomach, or duodenum within the upper GI tract.
20. Abbreviation for nonsteroidal anti-inflammatory drugs.
21. A digestive enzyme, this is activated at a pH of 2, and can cause mucosal damage.

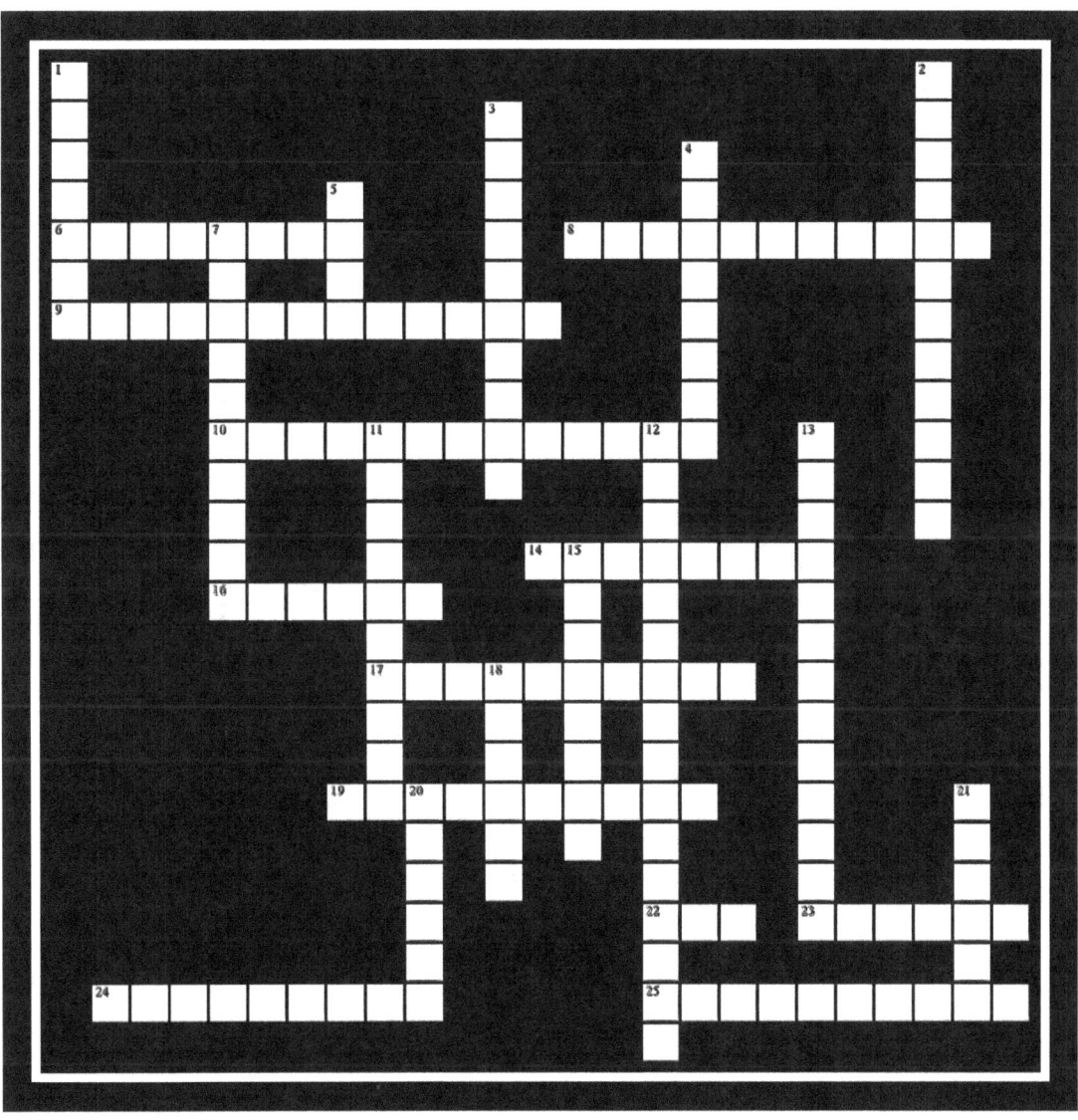

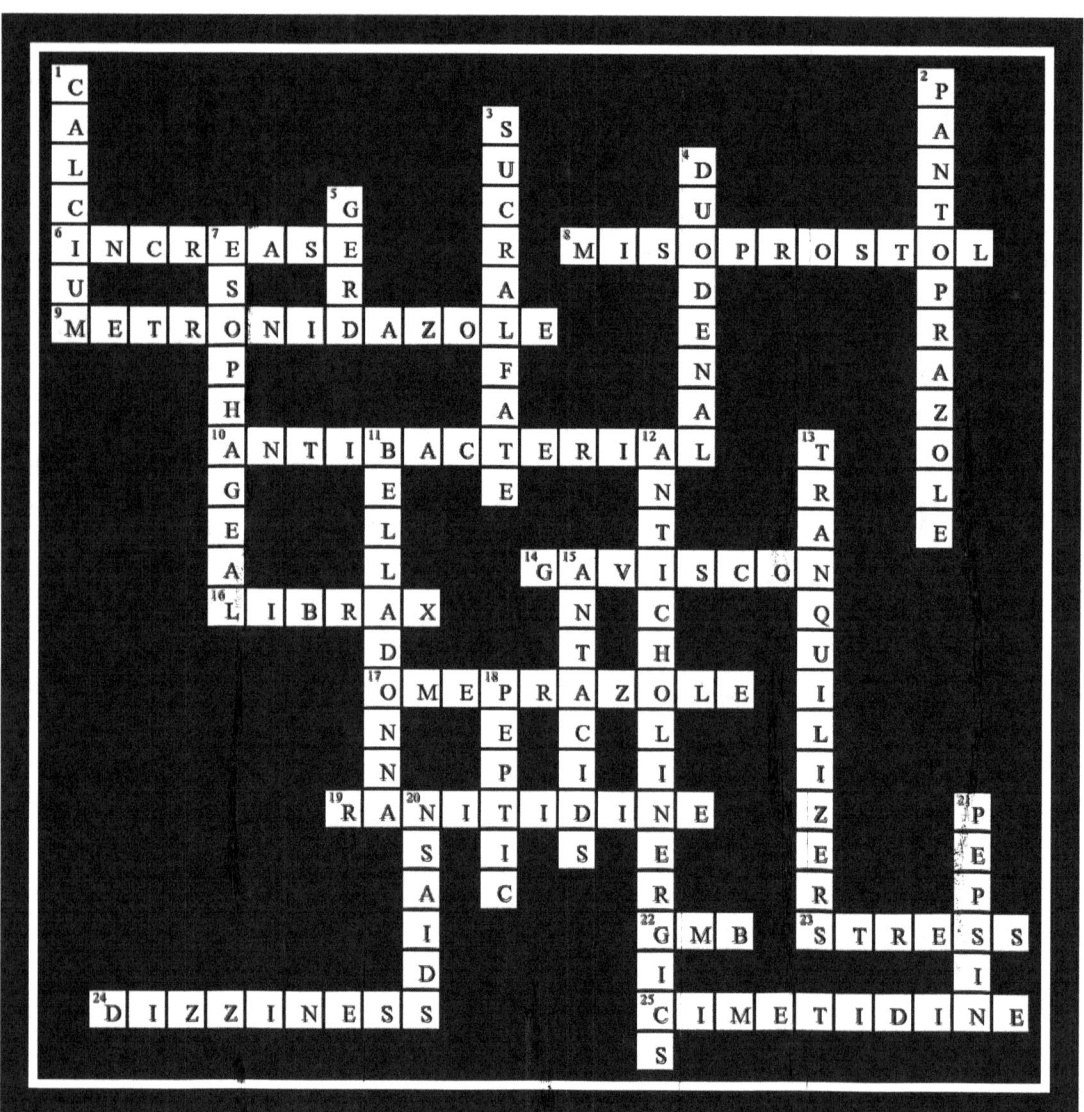

Pharmacology
Crossword Challenge
Gastrointestinal Agents
Antiulcer Drugs
Section XIII
Notes

Pharmacology
Crossword Challenge
Eye, Ear and Skin Agents
Eye and Ear Drugs
Section XIV

Across

5. Use of this herb is to be avoided in patients with glaucoma.

6. The term used to describe a local infection of eyelash follicles and glands on lid margins.

9. This is a combination of tobramycin and dexamethasone used in the treatment of fungal or viral infections of the eye.

10. Direct visualization of this membrane is recommended for ear irrigations.

11. These agents are used in open-angle glaucoma to lower the IOP.

14. Agents that paralyzes the ciliary muscle and thus the power of accommodation.

16. The generic name of this drug which may be used for patients sensitive to atropine sulfate.

17. This duct allows for passage of tears into the nose.

20. One contraindication in the use of mannitol is ___.

22. The generic name for Ceclor. This agent is a second-generation cephalosporin.

23. These agents are generally used pre- and postoperatively to decrease vitreous humor volume.

Down

1. Prostaglandin analogues are currently known to be effective in the treatment of this eye disorder.

2. The term used to describe an infection of the margins of the eyelids.

3. The term used to describe corneal inflammation.

4. The generic name for Viroptic, an antiinfective, used in the treatment of herpetic ophthalmic infections.

7. The term used to describe an infection of the vascular layer of the eye.

8. The generic name for Betoptic. A selective beta blocker used to decrease elevated IOP.

12. An agent that dilates the pupil.

13. This osmotic agent decreases volume of intraocular fluid to lower ocular tension.

15. The generic name for Natacyn Ophthalmic, used as an antifungal. May cause transient stinging.

18. The term used to describe an infection of the meiobomian glands causing blockage of the ducts.

19. The prostaglandin analogue more effective in African Americans than non-African Americans.

21. Another term for earwax.

24. Commonly used abbreviation for intraocular pressure.

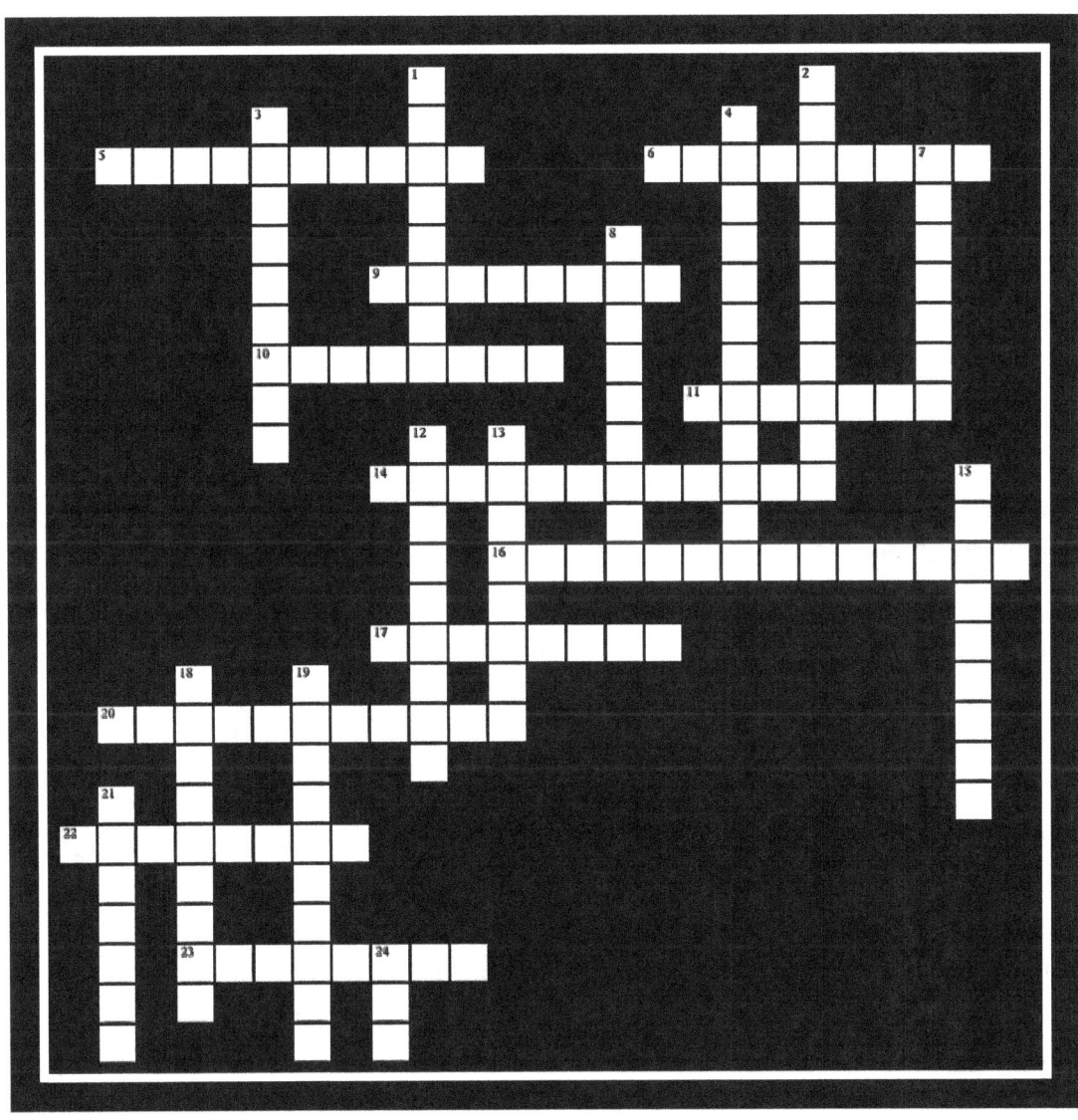

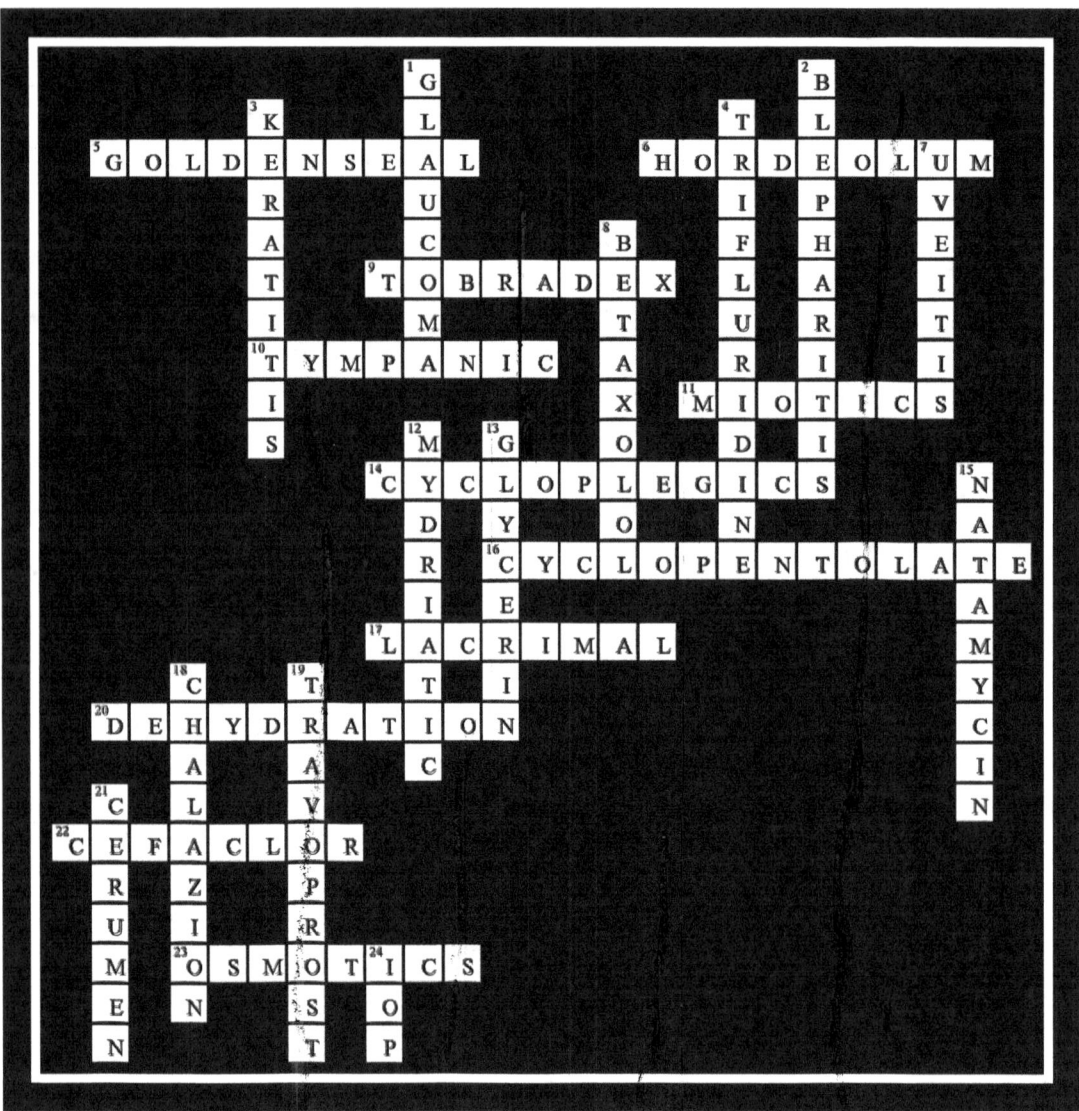

Pharmacology
Crossword Challenge
Eye, Ear and Skin Agents
Eye and Ear Drugs
Section XIV
Notes

Across

3. Flat skin lesions with varying colors.
4. The generic name for Rogaine. This agent may be used for treating baldness.
8. The generic name for Verr-Canth. An agent used to remove the common wart.
12. The generic name for Accutane. This agent is a derivative of vitamin A and used in treatment of severe cystic acne.
13. This agent, a sulfonamide derivative, is used as a topical, water-soluble antibacterial agent to prevent burn infection.
14. The term used to describe the absence or loss of hair.
16. Destruction of lesions or sealing off of blood vessels (usually of the skin, but also of available surfaces of mucous membrane) by monopolar high-frequency electric current.
18. Burns from heat are referred to as ___ burns.
20. The term used to describe a separation or loosening of the horny layer of the epidermis.
21. The commonly used abbreviation for psoralen and ultraviolet A.
22. This is a chronic skin condition characterized by erythematous papules and plaques covered with silvery scales.
24. The term used to describe raised, palpable skin lesions, less than 1 cm in diameter.

Down

1. Another term for contact dermatitis, ___dermatitis.
2. This is the drug agent of choice for treatment of patients with severe acne.
5. This NSAID may cause alopecia.
6. This drug agent is used to treat male-pattern baldness.
7. The commonly known trade name for silver sulfadiazine. This agent is used to prevent and treat sepsis in second- and third-degree burns.
9. This program which replaced SMART in 2005 uses a central database to track isotretinoin users.
10. These types of measure should be tried before drug therapy is initiated.
11. A hypersensitive reaction to a drug is caused by the formation of sensitizing ___.
15. The generic name for Cleocin. This agent is used for cases of moderate acne.
17. A full-thickness burn is referred to a ___ degree burn.
19. The generic name for Amevive. This agent is used in the treatment of severe, chronic plaque psoriasis. It inhibits T-cell activation.
23. Another name for verruca vulgaris

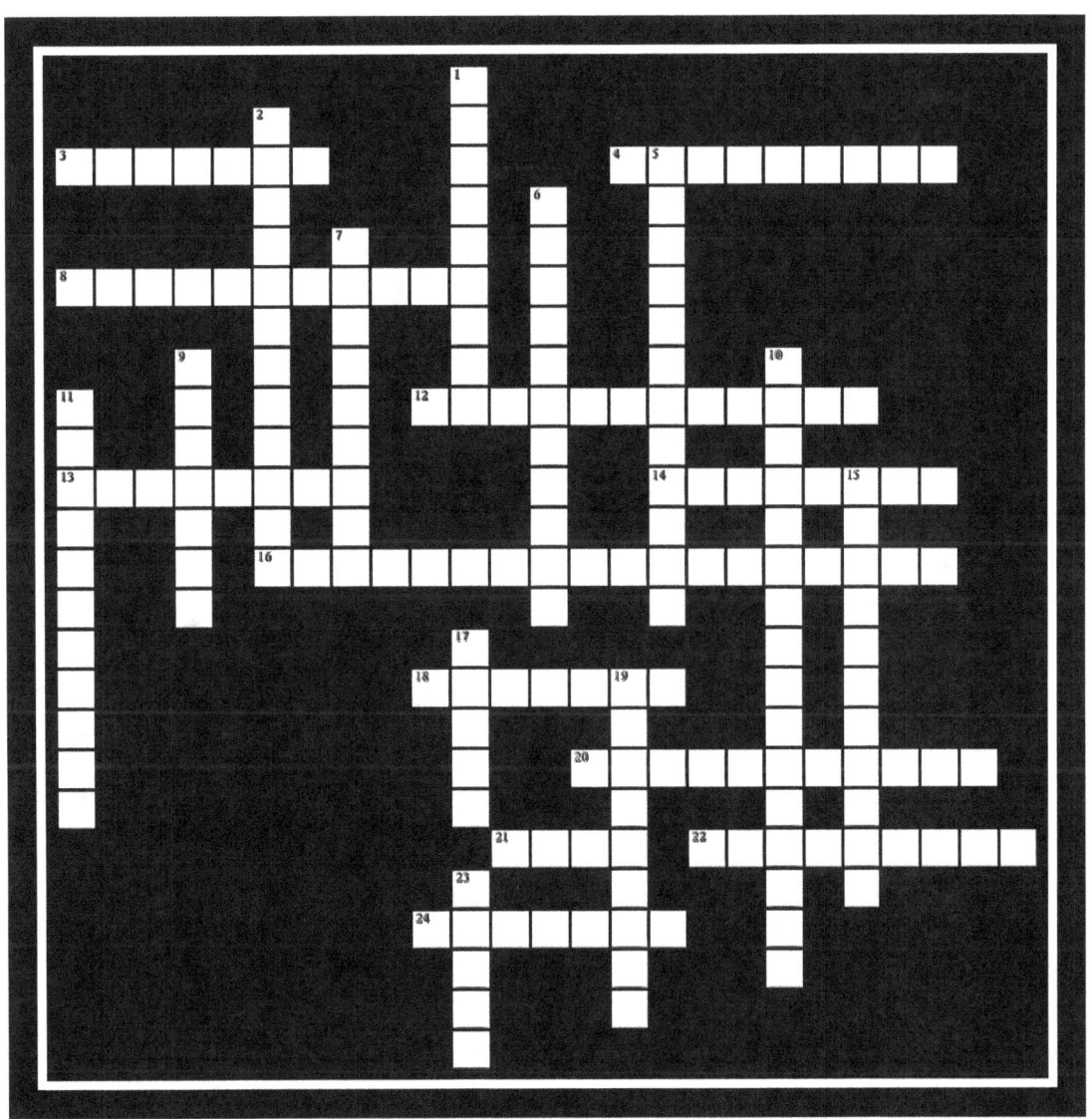

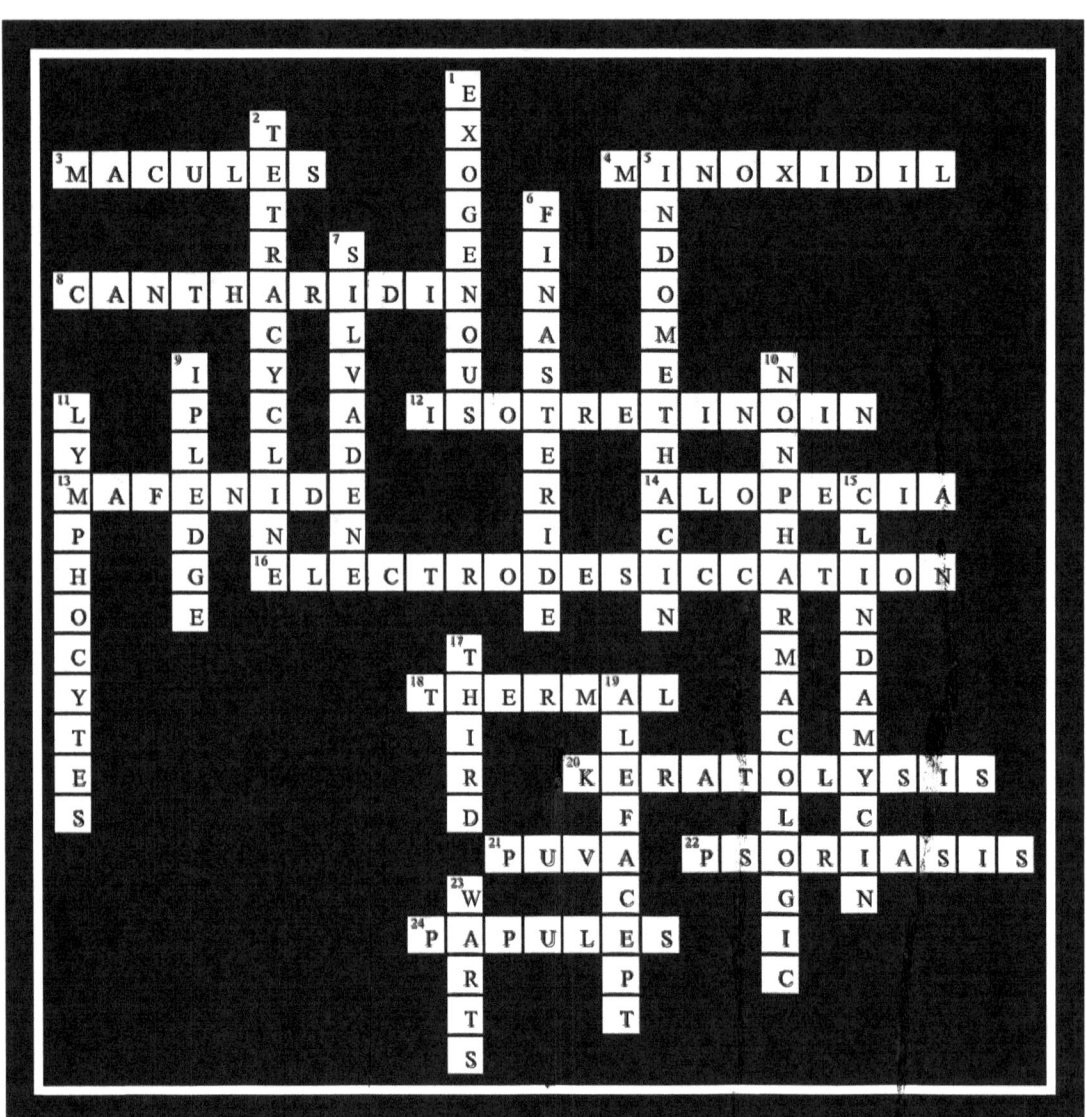

Pharmacology
Crossword Challenge
Eye, Ear and Skin Agents
Skin Agents
Section XIV
Notes

Across

5. Monitor for this adverse effect with patients taking levothyroxine.
9. Corticosteroids promote sodium ___.
11. Most of the wide variety of glucocorticoid drugs are frequently known as ___.
14. The generic name for Tapazole. This does not inhibit peripheral conversion to T4 to T3 and is 10 times more potent than PTU.
15. The paired adrenal glands consist of the adrenal medulla and the adrenal ___.
16. The generic name for Diapid. This drug is used for prevention or control of diabetes insipidus caused by insufficient ADH.
18. Secreted by the thyroid gland, regulates protein synthesis to stimulate mitochondrial oxidation.
20. Used in treatment of hyperthyroidism, to reduce the size and vascularity of the thyroid gland.
22. The term used to describe excessive growth after puberty.
23. The generic name for Rocaltrol. This drug is used to treat hypoparathyroidism and manage hypocalcemia in chronic renal failure.
24. This syndrome is a disorder resulting from increased adrenocortical secretion of cortisol.

Down

1. Commonly used abbreviation for antidiuretic hormone.
2. This hormone regulates calcium levels in the blood.
3. Its mode of action is the suppression of inflammation and adrenal function. It is readily absorbed from the GI tract and excreted primarily in the urine
4. The generic name for Lysodren. This is an antineoplastic agent that suppresses action of the adrenal gland. Used to treat Cushing syndrome.
6. This stimulates the adrenal gland to secrete corticosteroids.
7. This is a severe condition of hypothyroidism in the adult with symptoms of lethargy, edema of the eyelids and face, thickened and dry skin.
8. Another name for Graves disease.
10. The generic name for Synthroid. This agent is the drug of choice for replacement therapy in treatment of hypothyroidism.
12. These derivatives are the drugs of choice used to decrease thyroid hormone production.
13. The term used to describe the posterior pituitary gland.
17. Addison disease is caused by adrenal ___.
19. When this herb is taken with corticosteroids, central nervous system stimulation and insomnia may occur.
21. Commonly used abbreviation for adrenocorticotropic hormone.

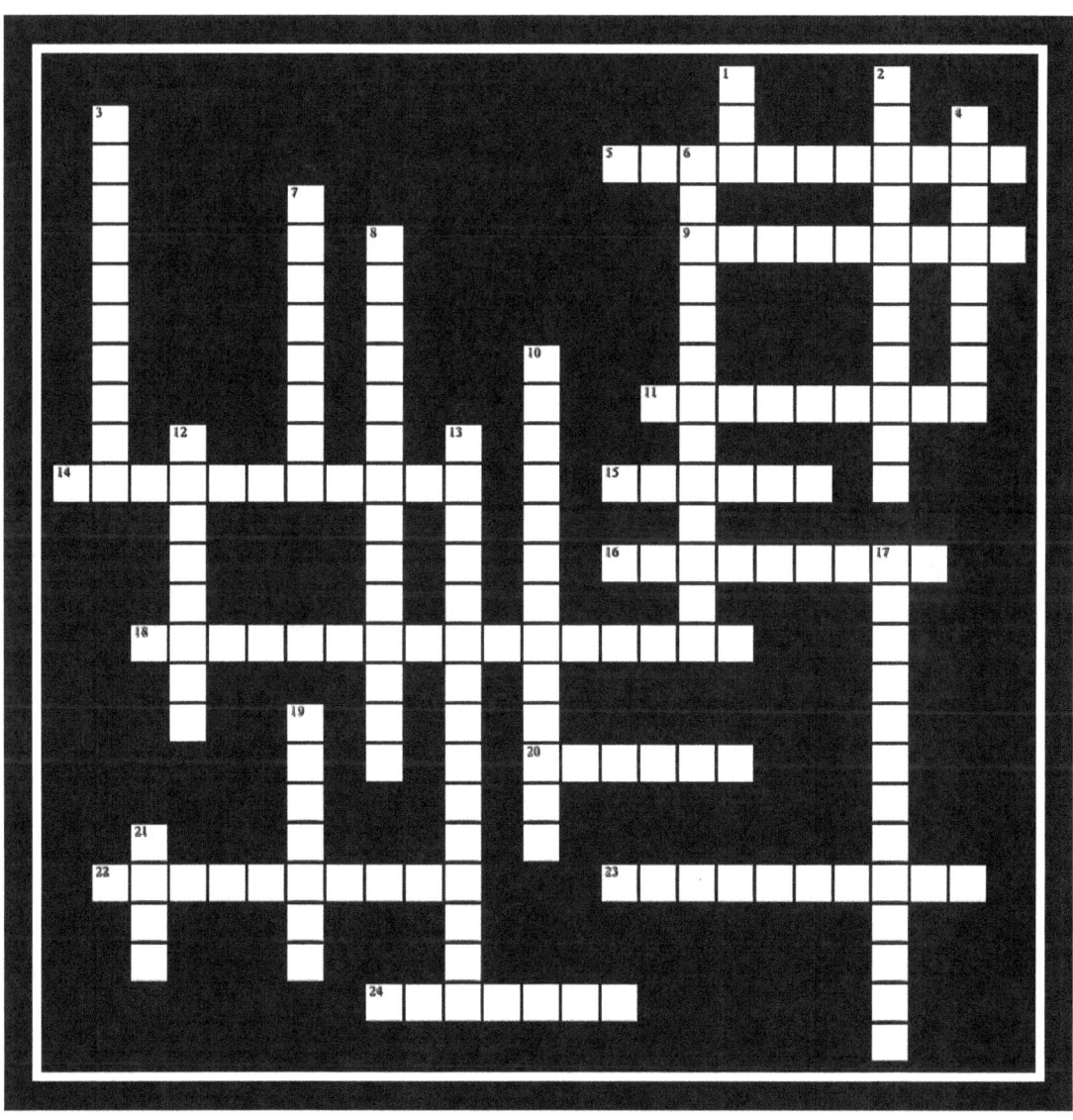

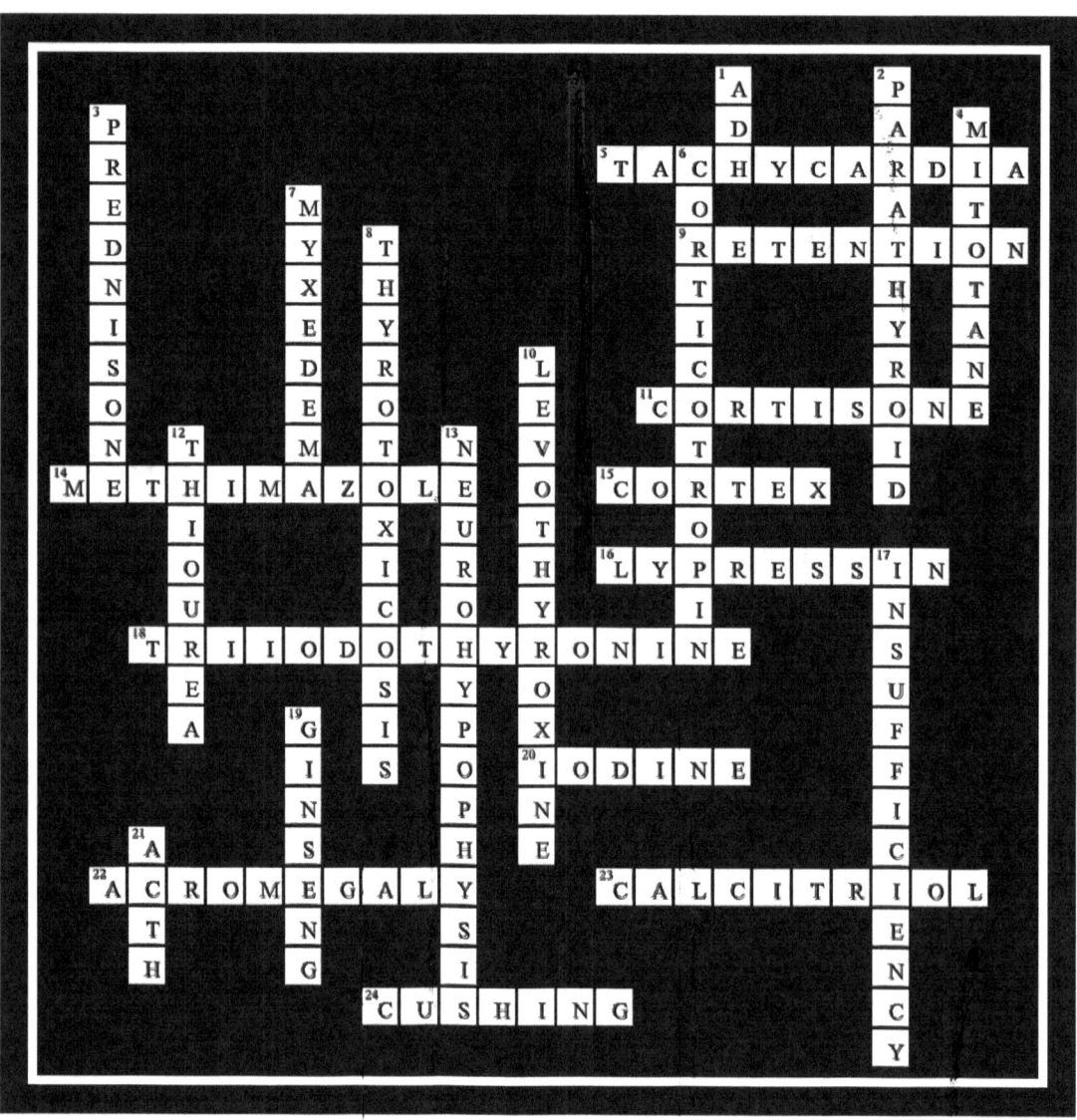

Pharmacology
Crossword Challenge
Endocrine Agents
Pituitary, Thyroid, Parathyroid, Adrenal Disorders
Section XV
Notes

Across

4. The generic name for Orinase, a first-generation, short acting oral antidiabetic.

6. Rapid- and short-acting insulins are in this type of solution.

9. Another term for oral antidiabetic drugs.

11. Commonly used abbreviation for non-insulin-dependent diabetes mellitus.

12. Insulin injections sites should be ___ to prevent lipodystrophy.

13. Intermediate-acting insulins are in this type of solution.

14. The term used to describe increased thirst.

16. The generic name for Avandia, a nonsulfonylurea oral antidiabetic.

17. A rapid-acting insulin.

21. The term used to describe tissue atrophy or hypertrophy.

22. The term used to describe increased hunger.

23. This is another term for injectable insulin.

Down

1. A condition in which the body uses fatty acids (ketones) for energy.

2. A possible adverse effect of taking glipizide.

3. Aspirin, oral anticoagulants, sulfonamides and some NSAIDS can increase the action of these agents.

5. These cells of the pancreas secrete units of insulin daily.

7. The insulin of a slaughtered animal which is most closely related to human insulin.

8. The generic name for Lantus, a long-acting insulin.

10. The generic name for Glucophage, a nonsulfonylurea oral antidiabetic

15. This compound acts by decreasing hepatic production of glucose from stored glycogen.

18. The generic name for Glucotrol, a second-generation oral antidiabetic.

19. The term used to describe increased urine output.

20. The generic name for Tolinase, a first-generation intermediate acting oral antidiabetic.

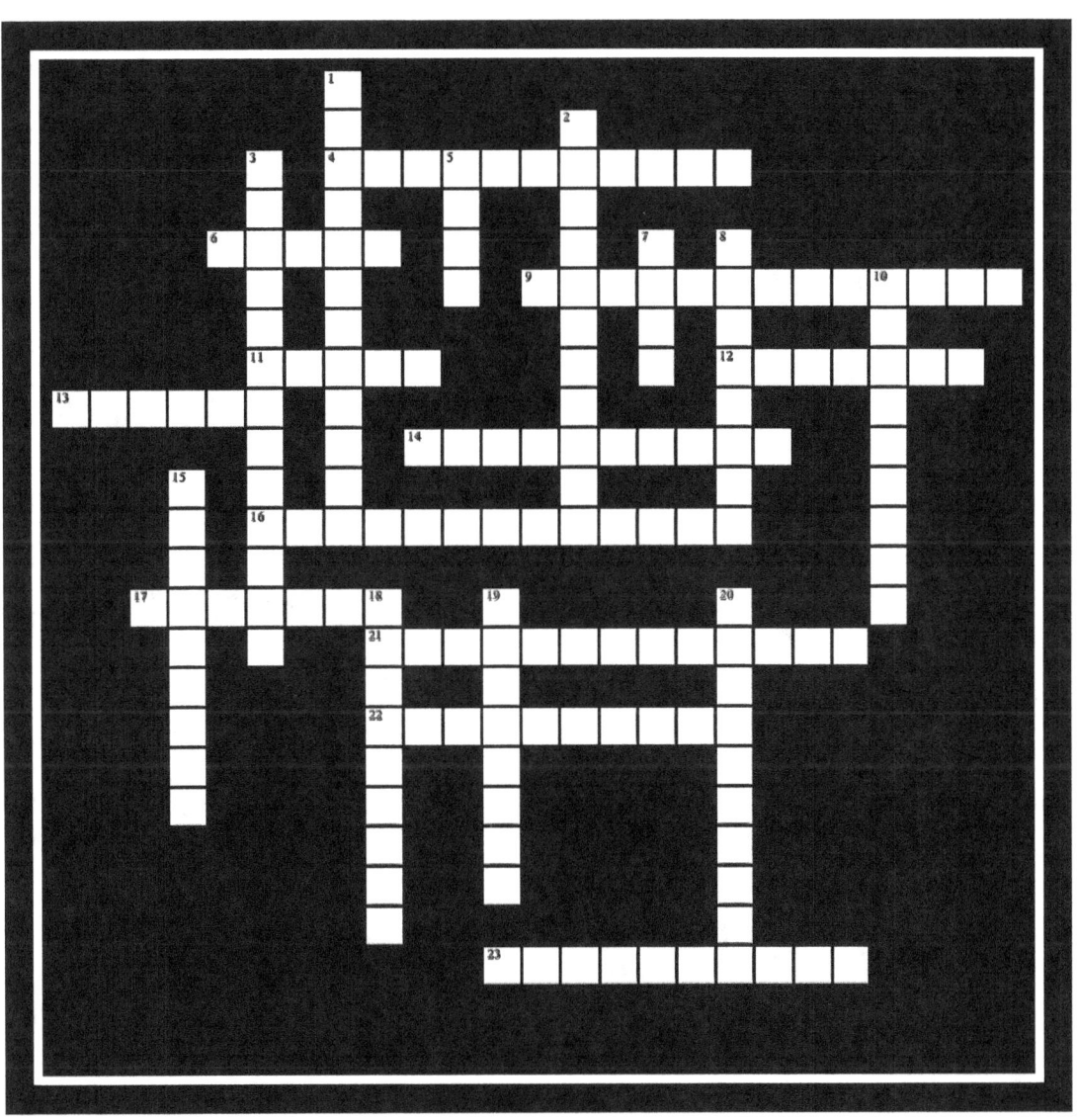

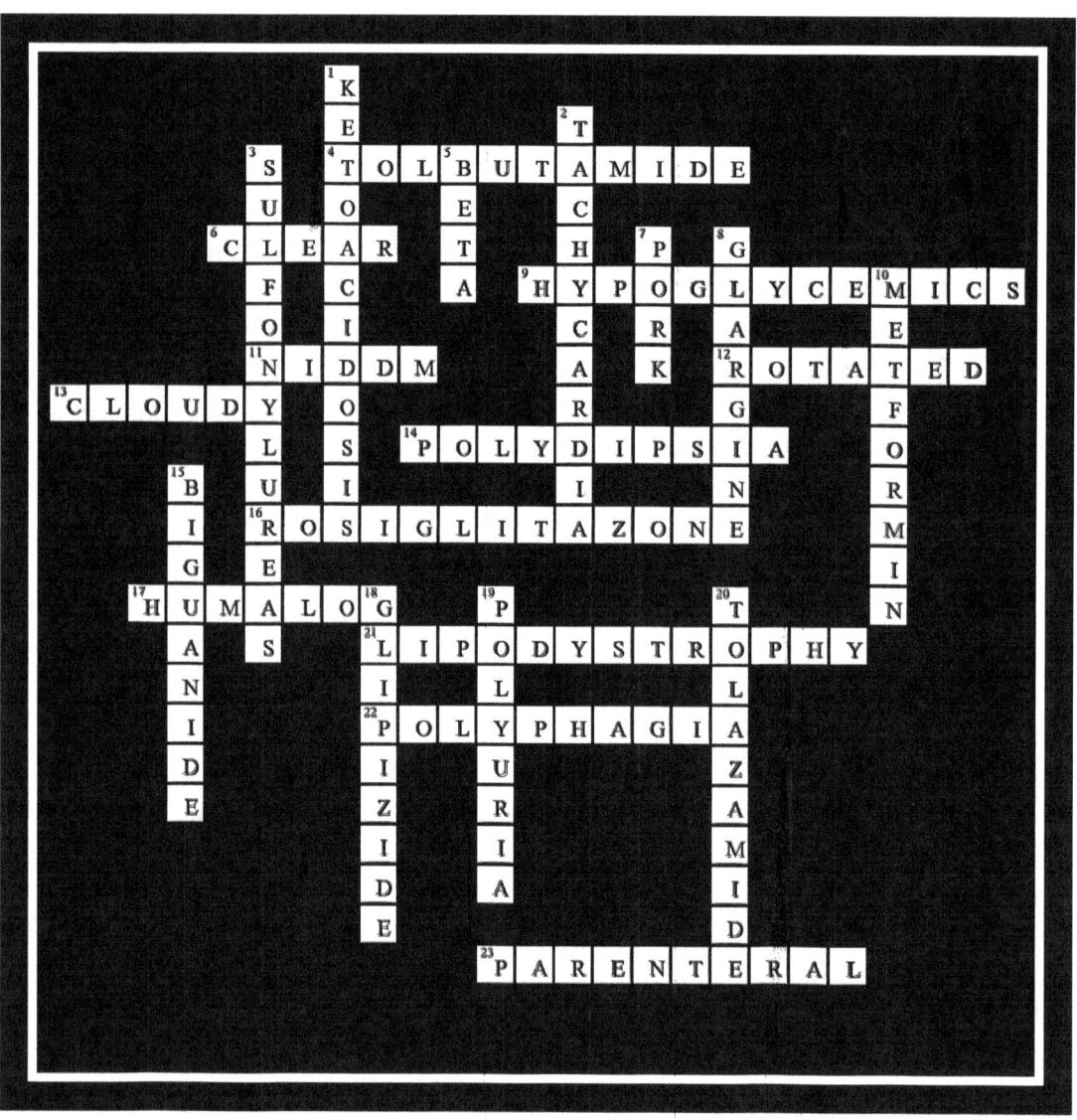

Pharmacology
Crossword Challenge
Endocrine Agents
Antidiabetics
Section XV
Notes

Across

5. This stool softener is used as first-line treatment for constipation.

6. This type of HTN may occur without proteinuria after 20 weeks of pregnancy.

7. Another term used to describe heartburn.

10. May be used for pain relief during all trimesters, short-term, for its antipyretic effects.

13. This type of drug therapy is used to decrease uterine muscle contractions.

15. These agents should not be taken with iron because they impair absorption.

16. This level of preeclampsia occurs with a BP increase of 160/110 on two occasions.

17. The generic name for Celestone. Corticosteroid. An injection given to mothers to prevent respiratory distress syndrome in preterm infants.

20. This type of administration of iron should be given through a plastic straw to prevent discoloration of teeth.

21. This syndrome is a severe sequela of preeclampsia and occurs in patients with gestational hypertension.

23. Taking this herb should be avoided during pregnancy as it is reported to decrease action of anticoagulants.

24. The generic name for Decadron. This agent has a rapid onset and shorter duration. Used as prenatal therapy for surfactant development.

25. One ounce of this substance twice a week may increase the risk of spontaneous abortion and may be responsible for FAS.

Down

1. The generic name for Apresoline. An antihypertensive for severe preeclampsia, causes arteriolar vasodilation.

2. This is the outer layer of the uterus.

3. The generic name for Reglan. Blocks dopamine receptors. Helps to control nausea and vomiting.

4. The generic name for Trandate. Used in cases of severe preeclampsia.

8. These methods should be tried initially for pain relief.

9. These are substances that cause developmental abnormalities.

11. Most commonly used abbreviation for preterm labor.

12. It is recommended that prenatal vitamins be taken with ___ .

14. Excess consumption of this substance may be toxic to the embryo.

18. The term used to describe new-onset grand mal seizures in a patient with pre-eclampsia.

19. This mild analgesic can inhibit the initiation of labor and prolong labor .

22. The most commonly used abbreviation for fetal alcohol syndrome.

Pharmacology
Crossword Challenge
Reproductive Agents
Female Reproductive, Pregnancy & Preterm Labor, Cycle I
Section XVI

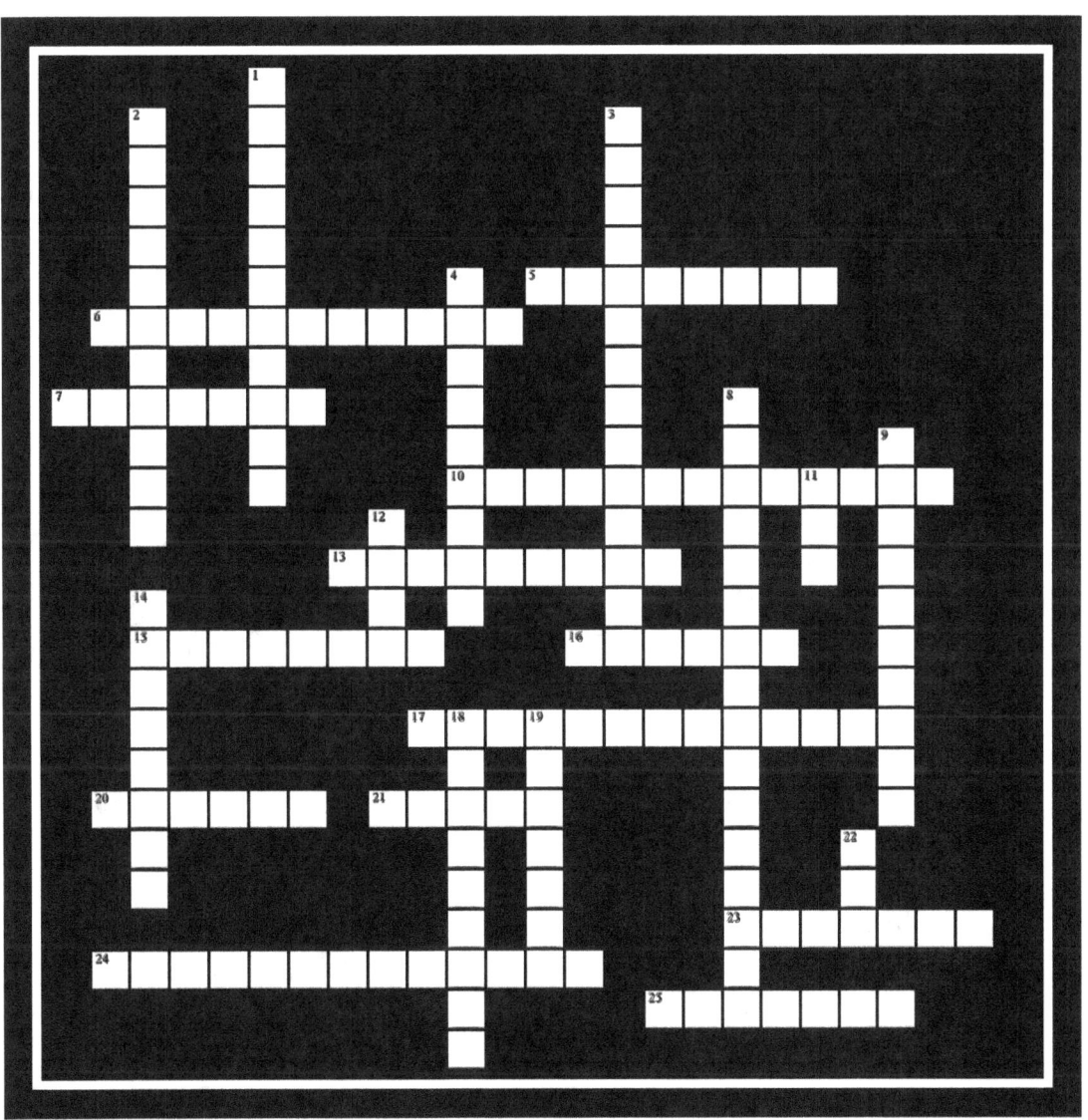

Pharmacology
Crossword Challenge
Reproductive Agents
Female Reproductive, Pregnancy & Preterm Labor, Cycle I
Section XVI

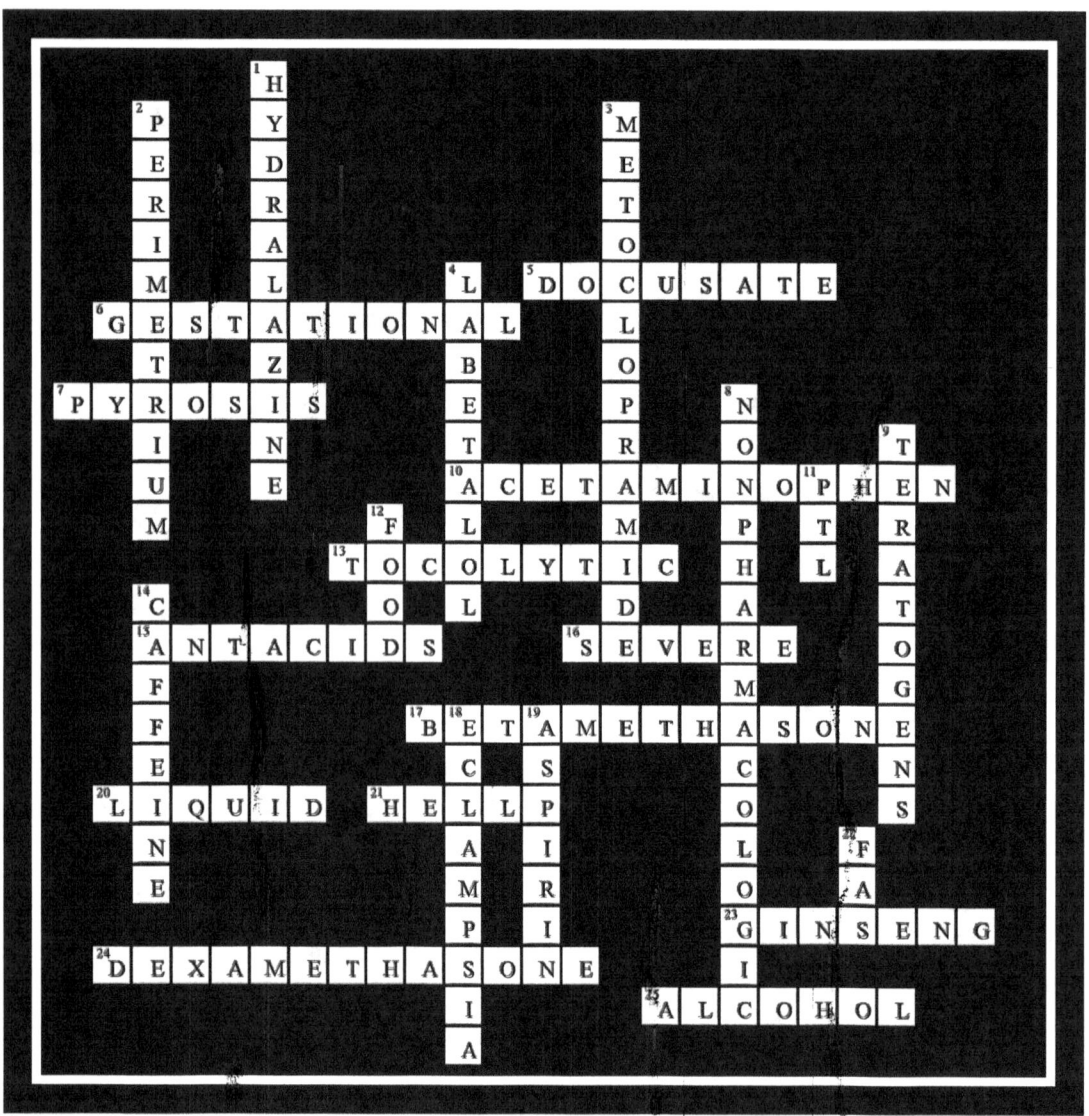

Pharmacology
Crossword Challenge
Reproductive Agents
Female Reproductive, Pregnancy & Preterm Labor, Cycle I
Section XVI
Notes

Across

5. This antacid is given to neutralize gastric contents.

7. This agent is used for cervical ripening.

10. A term used to describe uterine inactivity or hypotonic contractions.

11. This type of anesthesia is administered in the 2nd stage of labor, infrequently used.

12. The term used to describe discharge from the vagina of mucus, blood, and tissue debris, following childbirth.

13. The generic name for Pitocin, a uterotonic drug used to enhance contractility.

14. This is a condition which may be an indication for labor induction.

16. This agent is used in epidurals for cesarean section.

17. A nonpharmacologic measure for pain relief during labor.

19. The generic name for Survanta. Postnatal surfactant therapy for prevention of RDS.

21. Abbreviation for patient-controlled epidural anesthesia.

22. Nubain is administered at what point the uterine contraction.

23. The generic name for Seconal. This agent is used to decrease anxiety during the latent phase.

Down

1. The term used to describe a disproportion between fetal head and maternal pelvis.

2. A lipoprotein which reduces surface tension of pulmonary fluids.

3. With membrane stripping, there is a release of this substance.

4. Stimulation of effective uterine contractions once labor has begun.

6. This is an unfavorable fetal presentation.

8. This block is also referred to as a subarachnoid block.

9. The process of causing or initiating labor.

15. The generic name for Sublimaze. This is a narcotic agonist used for pain relief in labor.

16. The scoring system which helps to predict whether labor induction may be successful.

18. This is a sign of ergot toxicity which may include hallucinations and seizures.

20. This regional anesthesia is given after labor is well established.

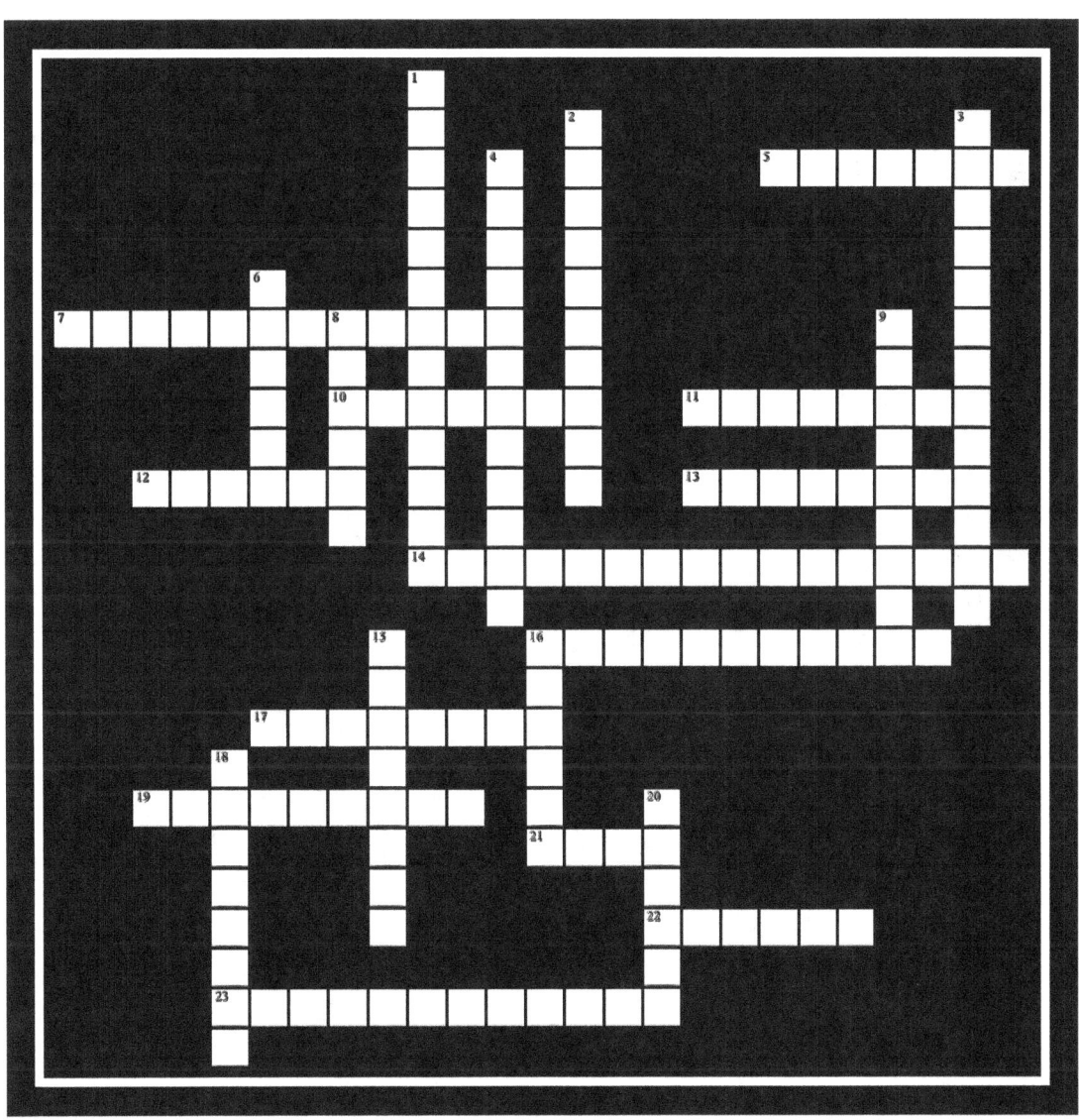

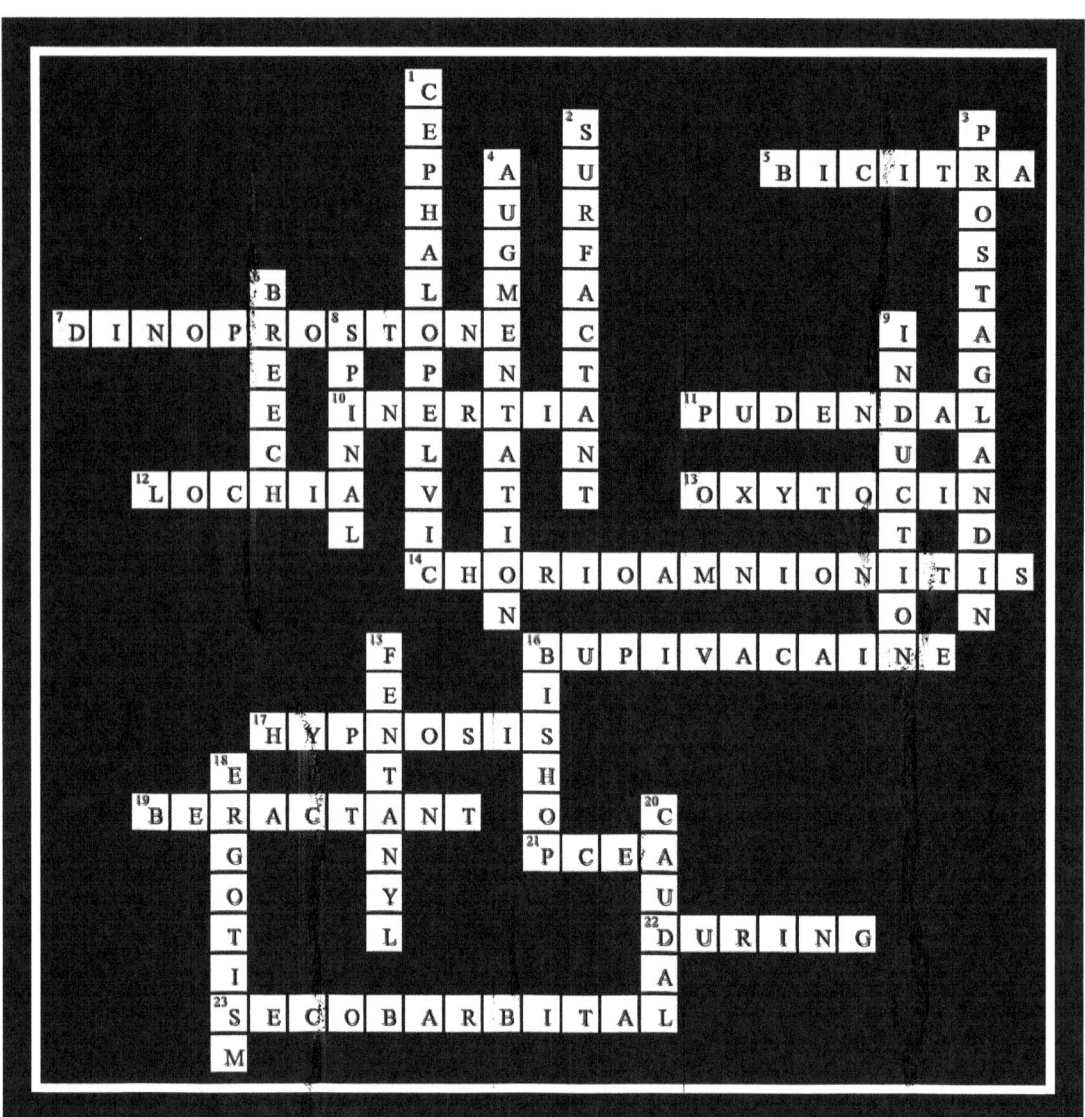

Pharmacology
Crossword Challenge
Reproductive Agents
Female Reproductive, Labor, Delivery, Cycle II
Section XVI
Notes

Across

3. Production and release of milk by mammary glands.

6. This ophthalmic ointment is administered to the newborn immediately after birth.

7. An allergy to this substance requires that you hold administration of MMR.

10. Maternal rubella is also known as this type of measles.

11. The generic name for Gax-X, an agent used to relieve flatulence.

13. This agent, vitamin K, should be administered prior to circumcision.

15. The period from delivery until six weeks postpartum.

17. Patients who receive this agent for pain should be assessed for bowel function and respirations.

19. These agents are used to decrease excess gas in the stomach.

20. This position is recommended to relieve hemorrhoidal pain and increase venous return.

22. Meruvax is the vaccine, is given for ___ .

23. This agent is prescribed for a patient with postpartum hemorrhage.

Down

1. This is one side effect with using bisacodyl suppositories.

2. This agent may be sprayed onto the perineum to relieve pain.

4. Motrin 800 mg t.i.d. is given as a routine medication order for vaginal delivery postpartum and typically is known as a ___ order.

5. A trade name for human D immunoglobulin.

6. A term used to describe an incision to enlarge the vaginal opening.

8. The term used to describe death of tissue caused by disease or injury.

9. The generic name for Senokot which is used as a stimulant laxative.

12. This topical corticosteroid aerosol foam may relieve pain from hemorrhoids.

14. These analgesics require ongoing assessment for GI bleeding.

16. This type of suppository should not be used by patients with 4th-degree perineal laceration.

18. The acronym for redness, ecchymosis, edema, discharge and approximation.

20. It is not recommended to use this cleanser on sore or cracked nipples.

21. This herbal supplement is not recommended during lactation.

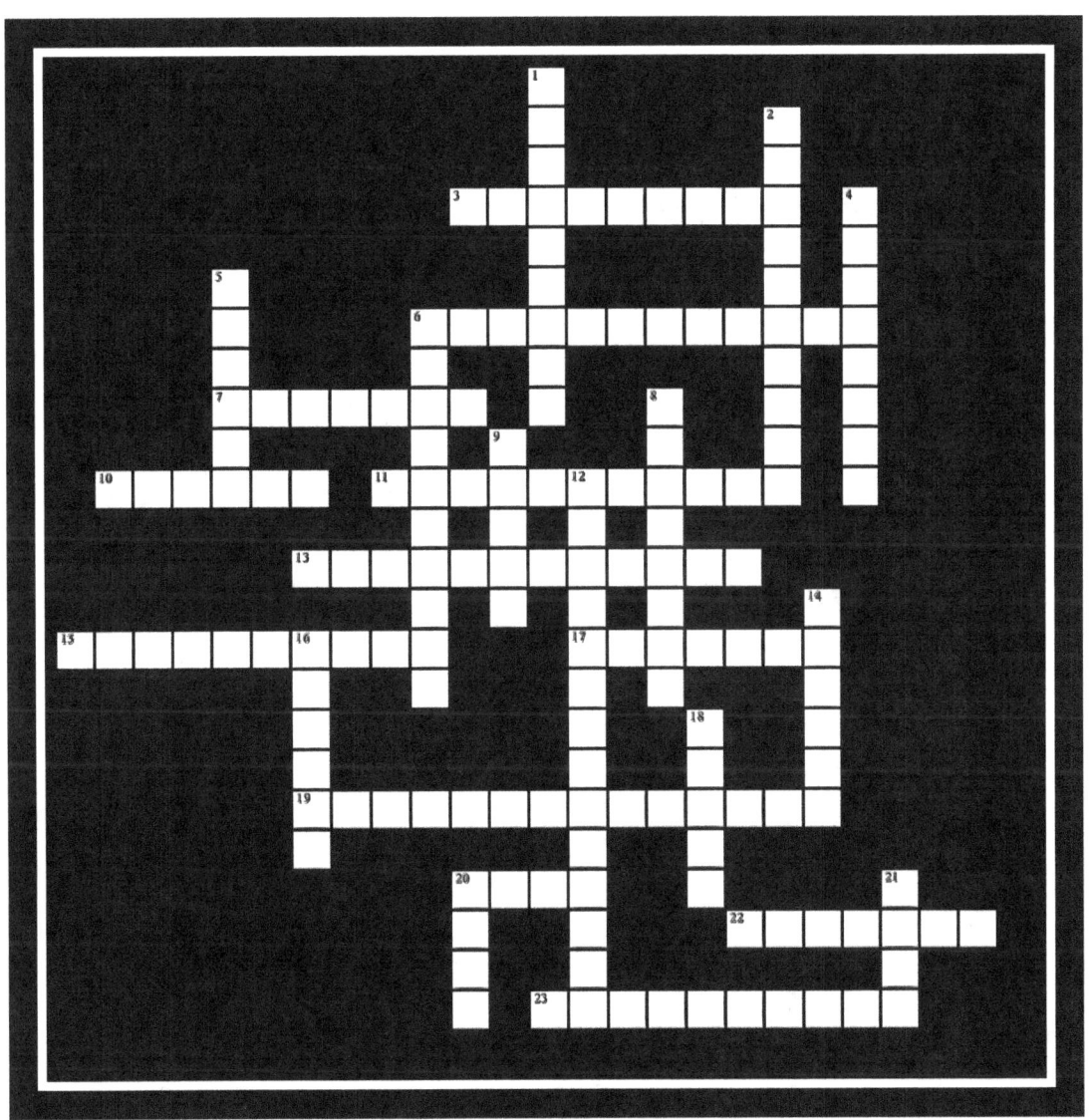

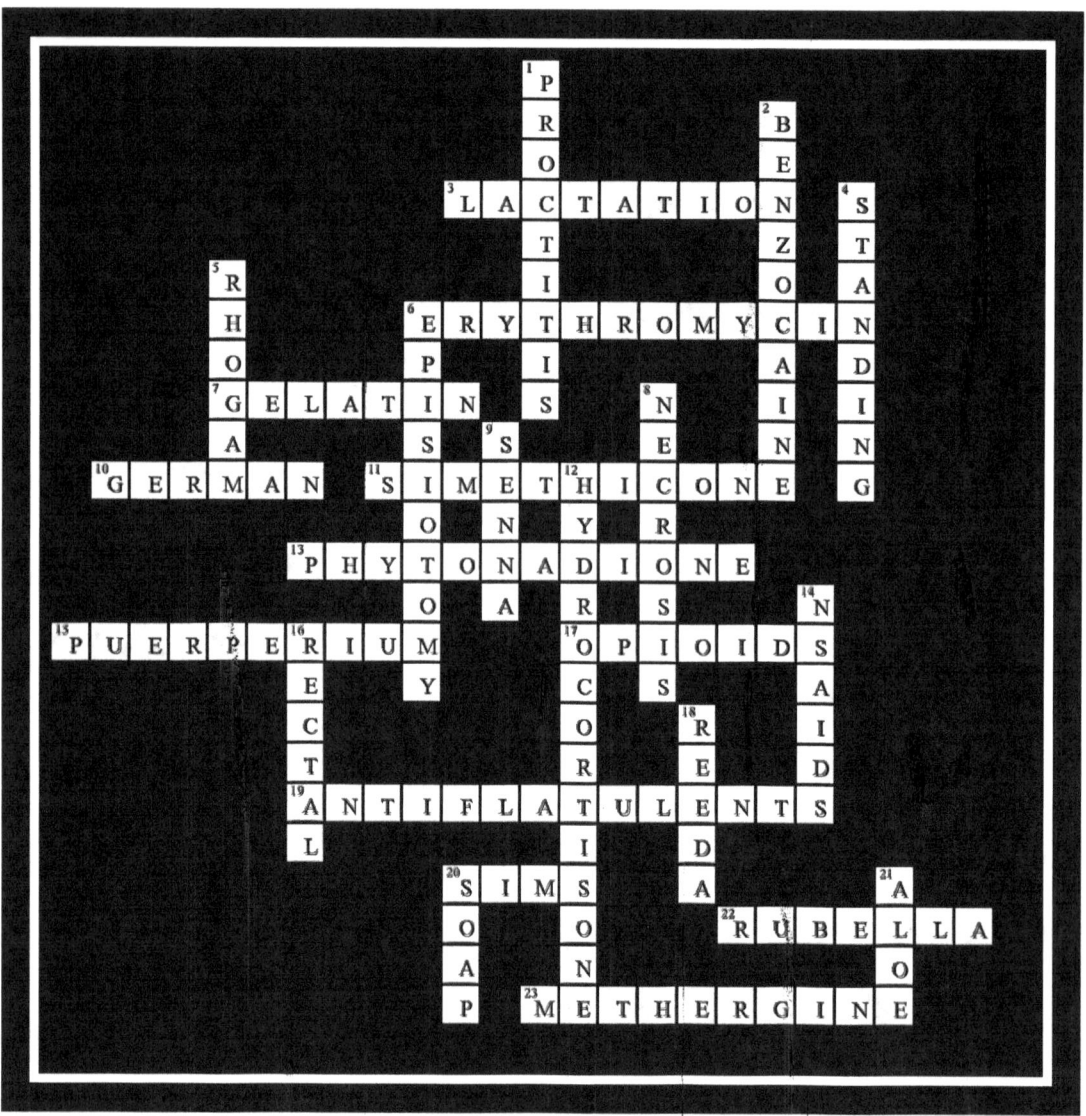

Pharmacology
Crossword Challenge
Reproductive Agents
Postpartum & Newborn Agents
Section XVI
Notes

Pharmacology
Crossword Challenge
Reproductive Agents
Women's Health & Reproductive Disorders
Section XVI

Across

2. Commonly used abbreviation for selective estrogen receptor modulator.
5. This drug is a pituitary gonadotropin inhibitory agent.
7. Extended-cycle regimen pills always have a start day on this day of the week.
9. The most prevalent treatment for relief of vasomotor symptoms and vaginal dryness.
10. PMS occurs in a repetitive regular pattern during this phase.
14. The condition used to describe the abnormal location of endometrial tissue outside the uterus in the pelvic cavity.
16. The name of the contraceptive that, if taken more than 3 hours late, a back-up contraceptive should be used for 48 hours.
17. This is the name of the first oral contraceptive with progestin to reduce water retention.
19. This device is 2 inches in diameter, inserted into the vagina, and releases estrogen.
21. This is the name of an elastomer ring inserted into the vagina where it releases estradiol for 3 months.
22. The name of the the first chewable birth control pill.

Down

1. This device is inserted into the vagina and releases copper which interferes with sperm motility and fertilization.
3. The generic name for Evista which is a selective estrogen receptor modifier that increases bone mineral density.
4. This combination type fixes the amount of estrogen throughout the cycle.
6. Hormones for treating symptoms of menopause and decreasing risks of cardiovascular disease in postmenopausal women.
8. The term used to describe painful, sexual intercourse.
10. This is the name of the first continuous-dose oral contraceptive pill to be FDA approved.
11. A long-acting injectable progestin, requires only one injection every 3 months.
12. This syndrome comprises a collection of varied physical, emotional and behavioral symptoms.
13. Oral contraceptives act by preventing ___.
15. This device is a single implant containing progestin and is an alternative method of contraceptive.
18. Most common type of combination product.
20. The first and only vaginal ERT to treat moderate-to-severe hot flashes, inserted into the upper vagina for 3 months.

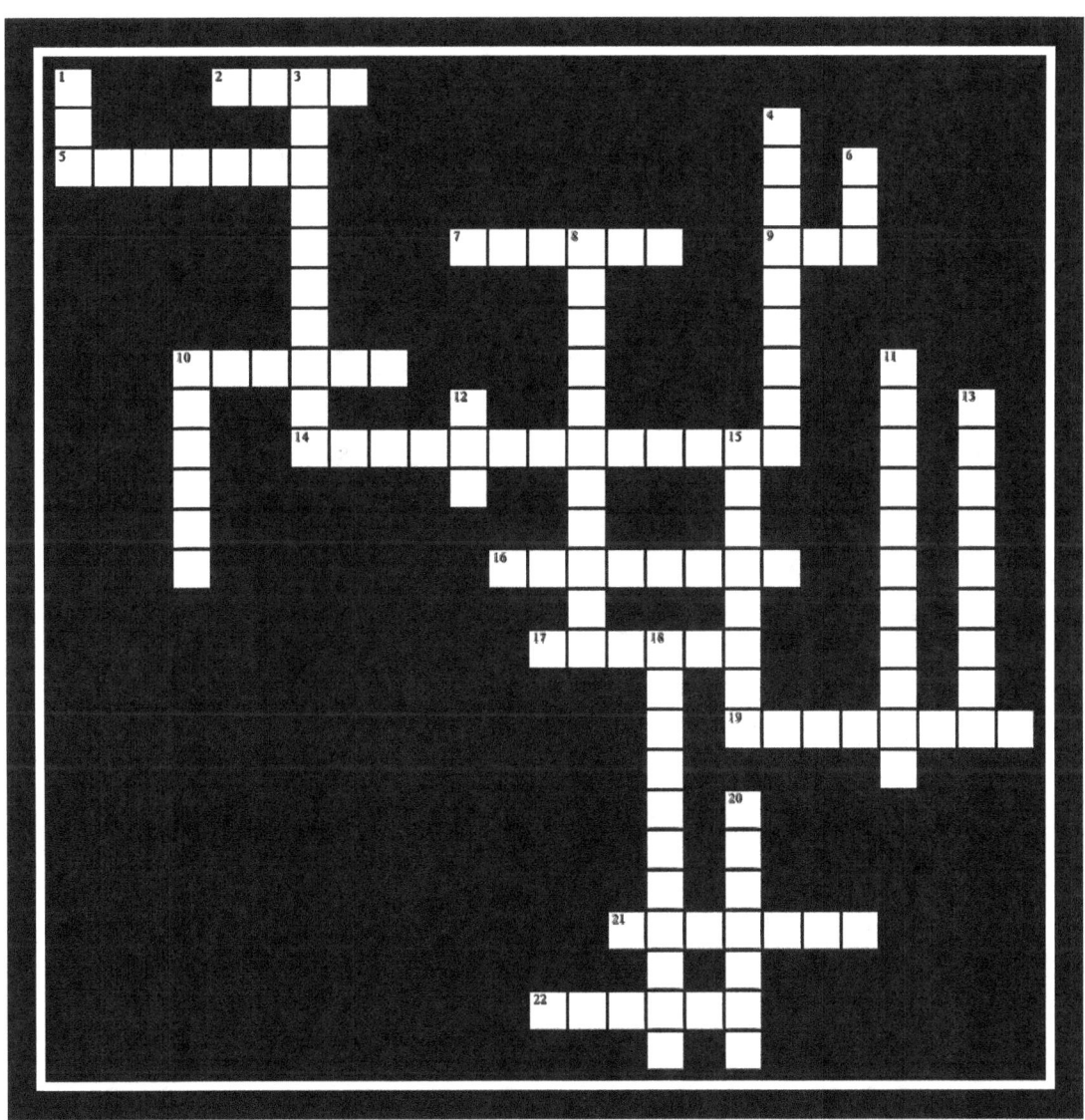

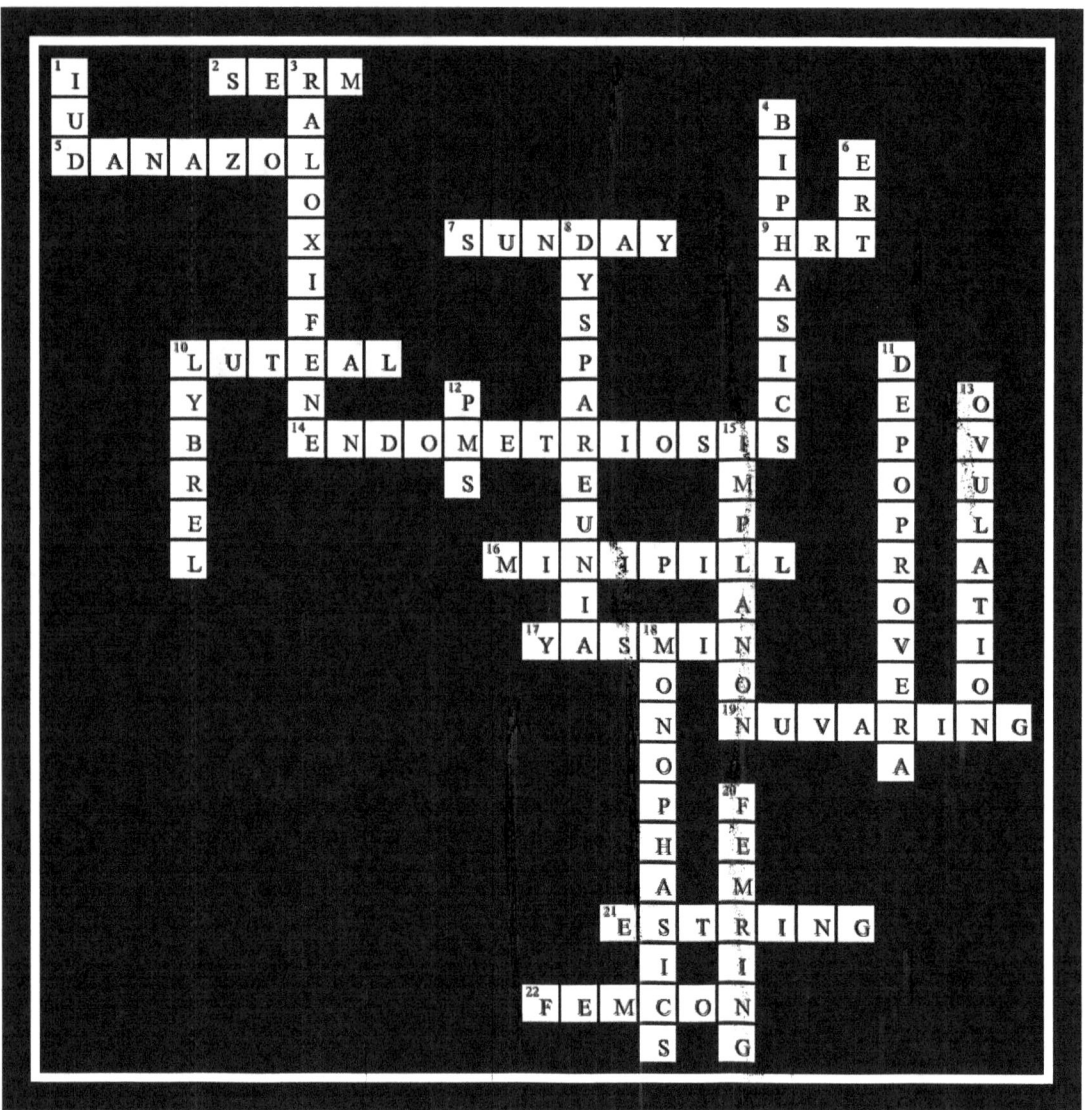

Pharmacology
Crossword Challenge
Reproductive Agents
Women's Health & Reproductive Disorders
Section XVI
Notes

Across

2. The term used to describe breast swelling or soreness.
8. The generic name for Oxandrin, an anabolic steroid given for delayed growth/puberty.
9. Transdermal testosterone patches should be applied to ___ area of the skin.
10. A term used to describe growth of facial hair and vocal huskiness.
13. This steroid inhibits conversion of testosterone to dihydrotestosterone.
17. A term used to describe plant-derived compounds.
19. The generic name for Cardura which is used in the treatment of BPH.
20. A condition in which there is a deficiency of thyroid hormone.
21. This dysfunction is characterized by persistent inability to attain or maintain a satisfactory erection.
22. Men receiving this agent show elevations in plasma LH and testosterone.
23. The term used to describe increased hair growth.
24. This condition is a common symptom of an enlarged prostate.

Down

1. Also known as "Spanish Fly" has been reported to cause bladder and urethral irritation and possible permanent penile damage.
2. The commonly used abbreviation for gonadotropin-releasing hormone.
3. The term used to describe undescended testis
4. These type of steroids are synthetic derivatives of testosterone developed to maximize effects of androgens.
5. With this disease, there is a deficit of both cortisol and mineralocorticoid aldosterone.
6. Commonly used abbreviation for phosphodiesterase. These inhibitors facilitate erections by enhancing blood flow to the penis.
7. The generic name for Halotestin, a synthetic androgen, given for androgen deficiency.
11. These are androgen antagonists. They block the synthesis of androgens.
12. This is one of several drugs considered as organic nitrates.
14. The generic name for Cialis. Used in treatment of erectile dysfunction.
15. This natural product has been used with positive effects when taken to improve erections.
16. This dysfunction is described as an impaired ejection of seminal fluid from the urethra of the male.
18. This is a common side effect when taking drugs to treat BPH.

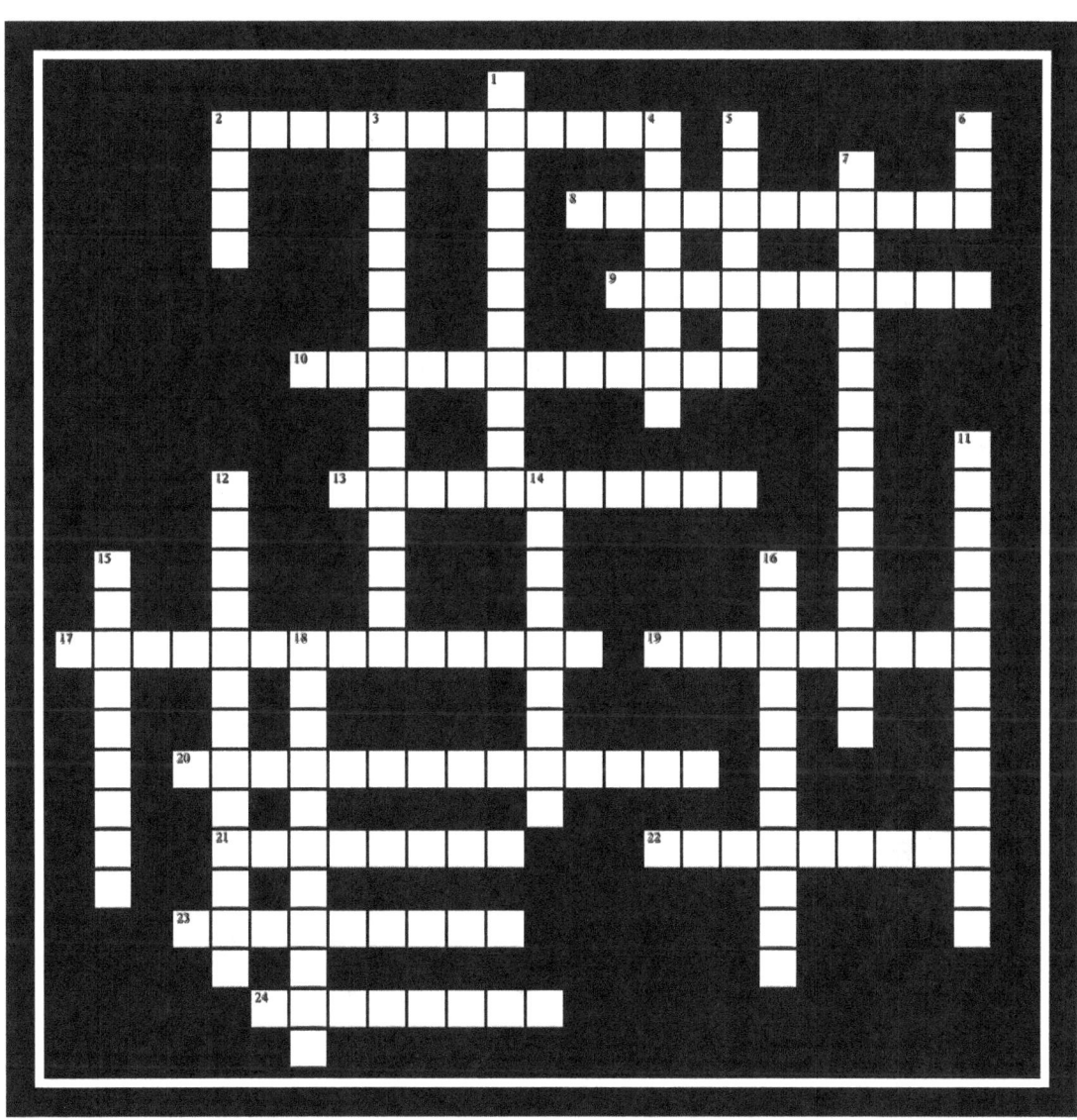

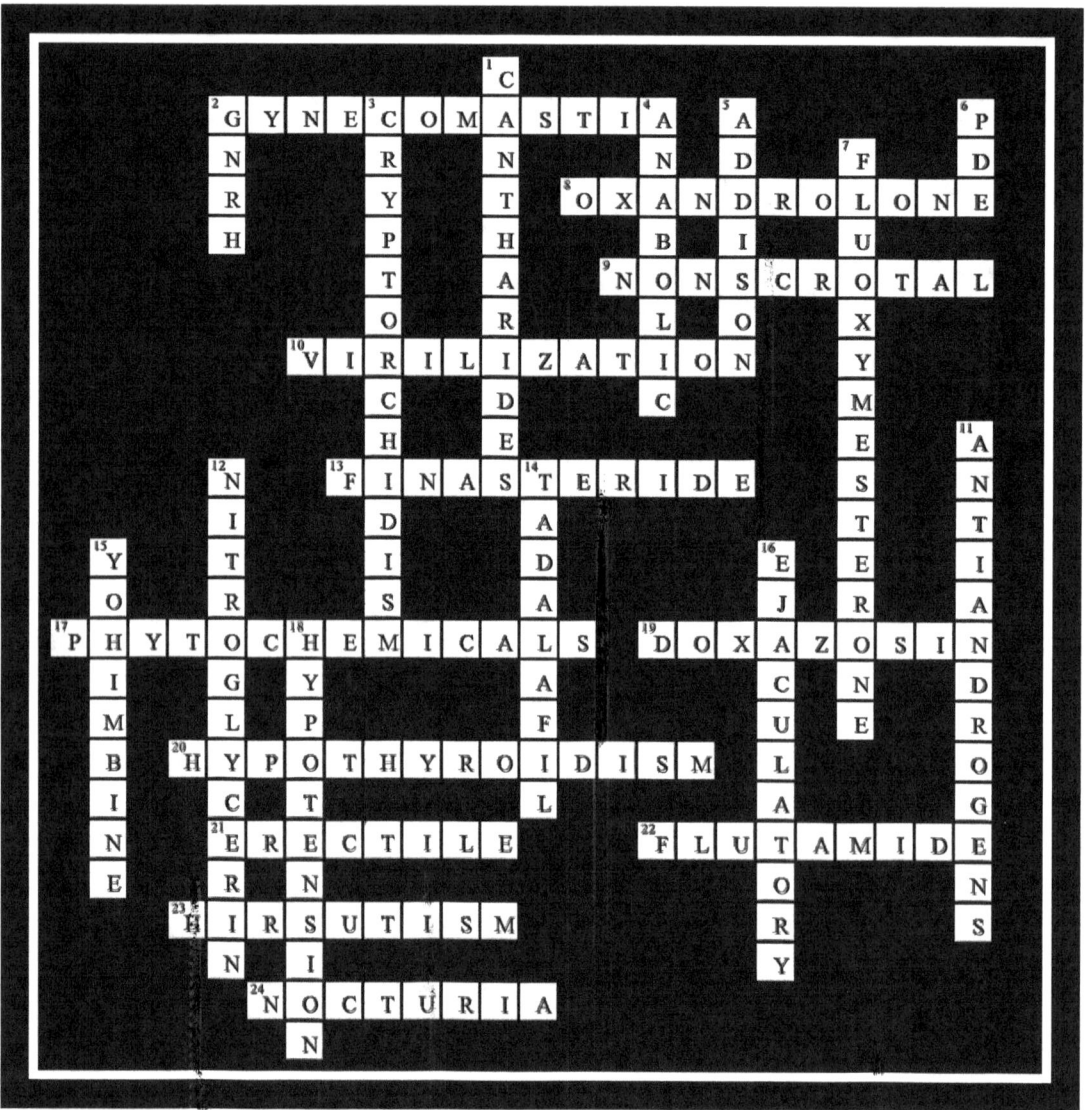

Pharmacology
Crossword Challenge
Reproductive Agents
Men's Health
Section XVI
Notes

Across

3. This is the term to describe the route of administration when a tablet is held inside the cheek until it dissolves.

5. An acute and chronic infectious disease caused by the bacterium Treponema pallidum and transmitted by direct contact, usually through sexual intercourse.

7. This therapy is used in the treatment of genital warts.

10. This drug is administered in the treatment of genital herpes simplex.

11. This term describes an infection of the testicles.

13. A term used to describe an infection of the epididymis.

15. The term used to describe a subnormal concentration of spermatozoa in the penile ejaculate.

16. This transmission occurs when a fetus or neonate is infected by the mother.

20. The generic name for Parlodel which is an ovulatory stimulant that normalizes prolactin levels.

21. Ceftriaxone is given as a primary therapy in the treatment of this STD.

22. The term used to describe intrauterine infection.

23. The inability to conceive a child after 12 months of unprotected sexual intercourse.

Down

1. This agent is given as primary therapy in the treatment of candidiasis.

2. This infertility affects couples who are unable to conceive after their first live birth.

4. The commonly used abbreviation for follicle-stimulating hormone.

6. This purpose of this exam is to evaluate fallopian tube patency.

7. This bacterial pathogen is transmitted predominately through sexual contact.

8. This pathogen causes Trichomonas

9. This vaccine is indicated for girls and women ages 9 to 26 for prevention of cervical cancer and genital warts.

12. Permethrin is used in the treatment of this condition.

14. A drug or other agent that causes abnormal prenatal development.

17. The generic name for Clomid which is an agent used as an ovulatory stimulant.

18. This cream rinse is applied as primary therapy in treatment of pubic lice.

19. Infections that are transmitted during sexual contact.

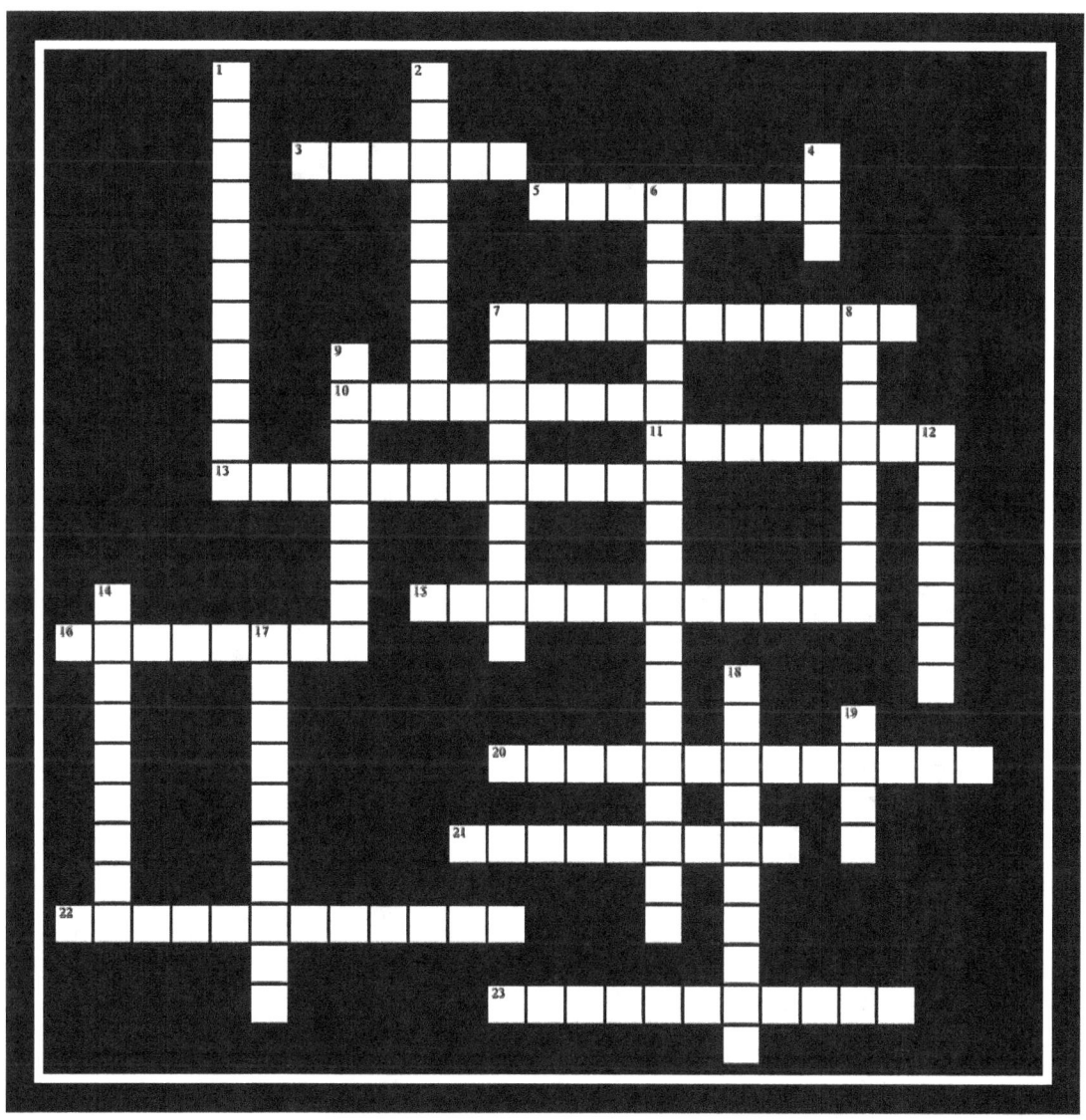

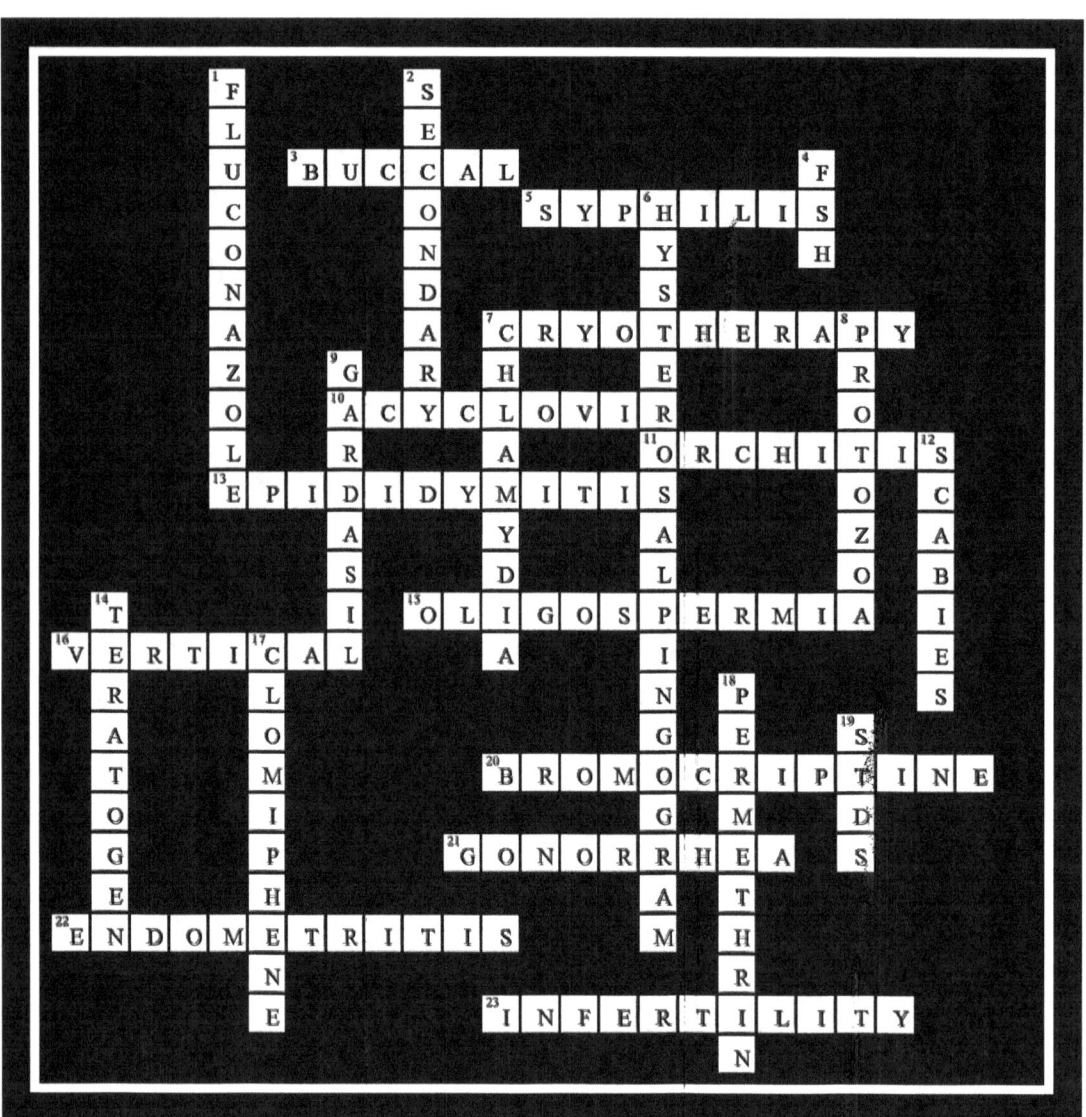

Pharmacology
Crossword Challenge
Reproductive Agents
Infertility and STDs
Section XVI
Notes

Across

1. This osmotic diuretic is used to treat cerebral edema and increased intracranial pressure.
4. The commonly used abbreviation for paroxysmal supraventricular tachycardia.
7. Naloxone is effective for this class of drug overdose.
8. This term describes the amount of blood returning to the right ventricle.
10. This sodium is an IV agent used to reduce arterial blood pressure in hypertensive crisis.
13. This beta-adrenergic drug is given to increase the heart rate.
16. The term used to describe that which passes out of a vessel into the tissues, said of blood, lymph, or urine.
19. This term is used to describe the hydrolysis of glycogen to glucose.
20. The term used to describe a low serum magnesium level.
23. This beta-adrenergic bronchodilator is used to reverse bronchoconstriction in anaphylactic shock.
24. This hormone is produced in the pancreas. It elevates blood sugar by stimulating glycogen break down.
25. This herb can inhibit the efficacy of furosemide.

Down

2. Shock. An allergic response of the most serious type
3. This gaseous element can be classified as a drug because it can have good and bad effects based on amount and manner administered.
5. This sulfate is indicated in the treatment of hemodynamically significant bradycardia.
6. This agent is the reversal agent for respiratory depression of benzodiazepine medications.
9. This drug is the first-line choice to treat PSVT.
11. This agent is classified as an antidysrhythmic. It is considered an alternative to amiodarone. It exerts a local anesthetic effect on the heart.
12. This sympathomimetic agent is often used to treat hypotension in shock not caused by hypovolemia.
14. This agent is considered the drug treatment of choice for angina pectoris.
15. This agent is used in the treatment of ventricular tachycardia and PVCs.
17. This agent is especially good for patients with impaired heart function who have atrial and ventricular dysrhythmias.
18. This is the term used to describe shock resulting from loss of blood or fluid volume.
21. This opiate antagonist reverses the effects of all opiate drugs.
22. This bicarbonate is prescribed to treat metabolic acidosis.

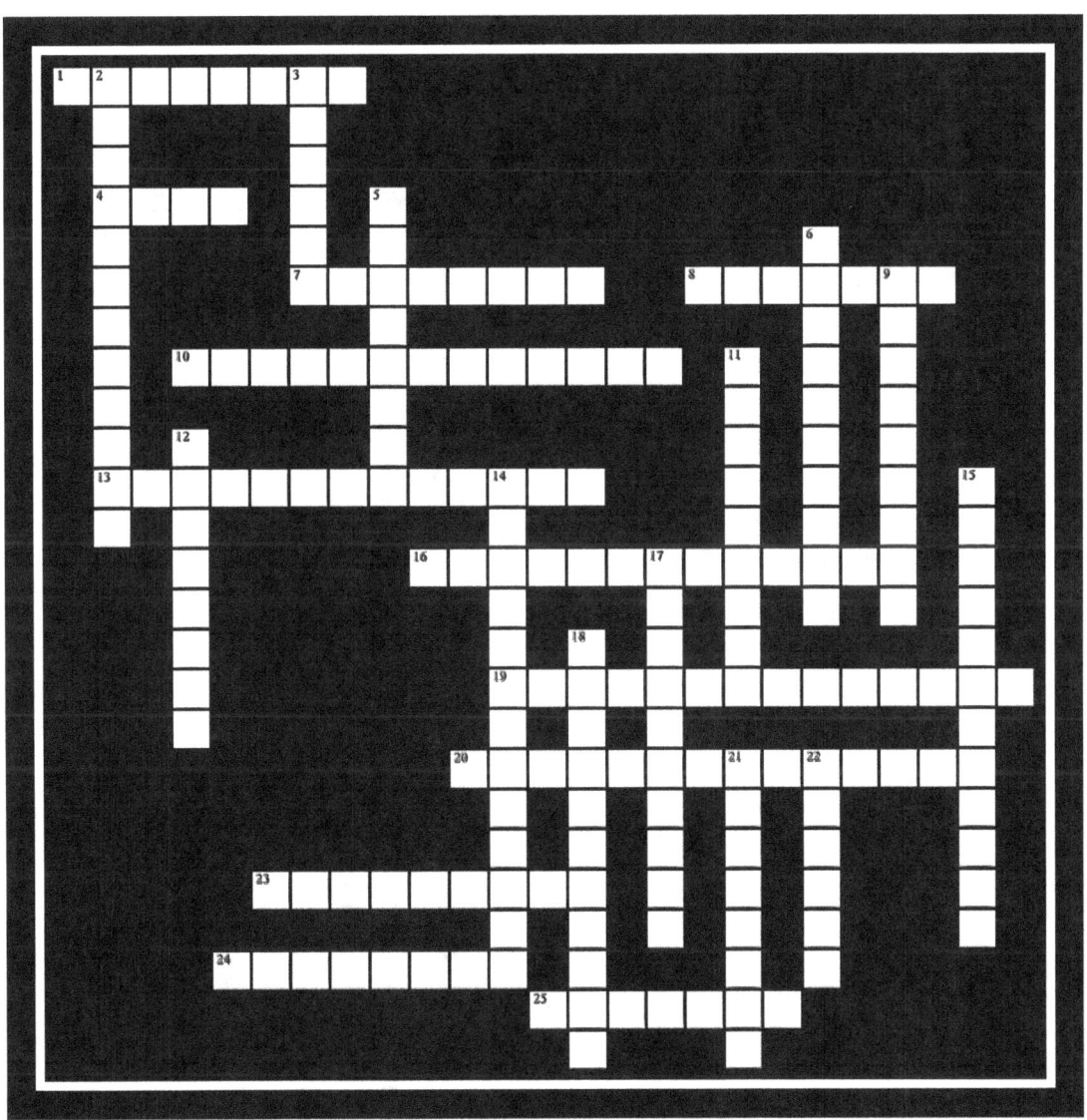

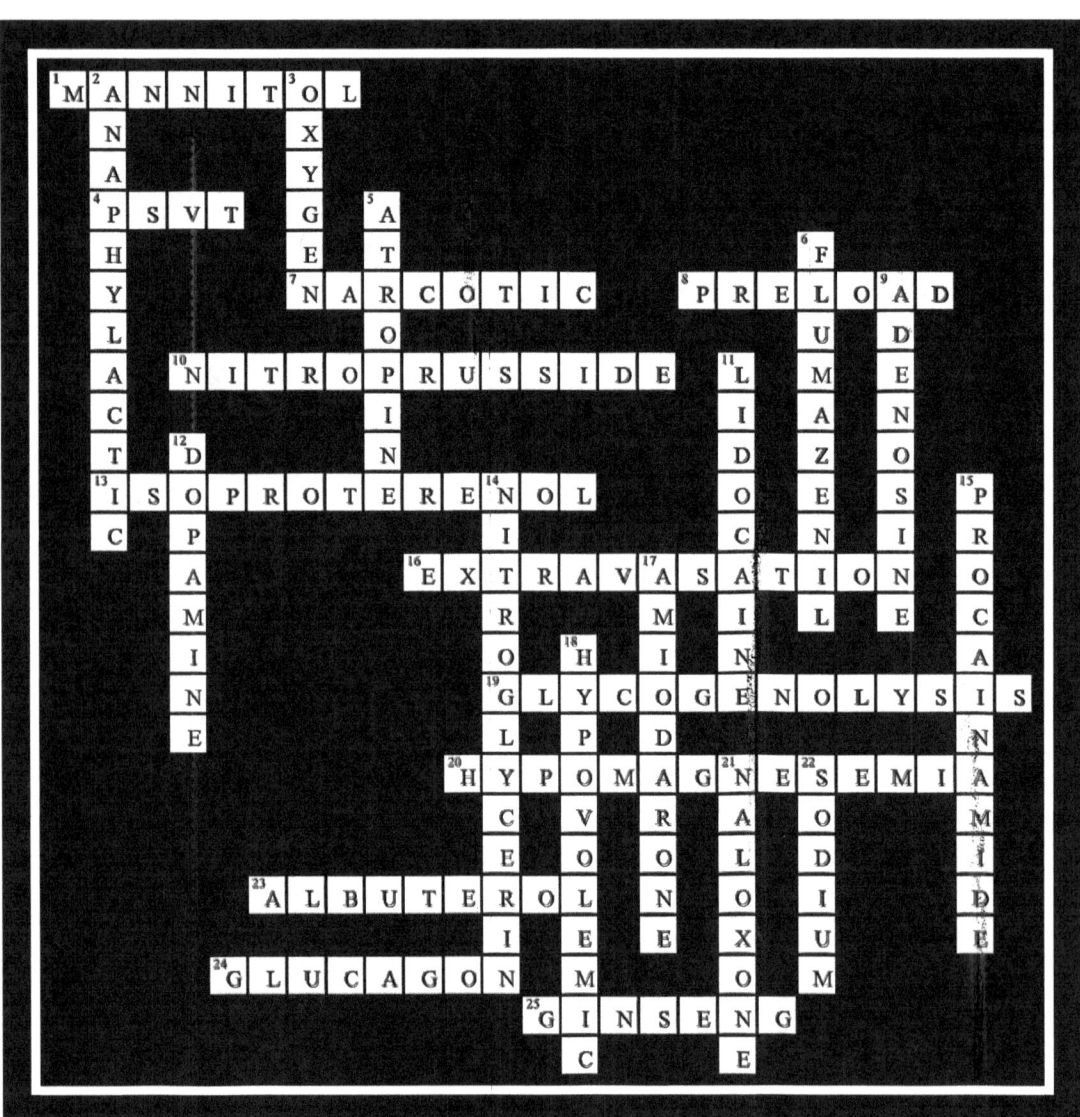

Pharmacology
Crossword Challenge
Emergency Agents
Section XVII
Notes

A

Abciximab
The generic name for ReoPro, used primarily for preventing re-occlusion of coronary arteries.

Absorption
The taking in, incorporation, or reception of gases, liquids, light or heat. The movement of drug particles from the GI tract to body fluids by passive absorption.

ACE
Commonly used abbreviation for angiotensin-converting enzyme.

Acetaminophen
May be used for pain relief during all trimesters, short-term, for its analgesic / antipyretic effects. This drug should be used instead of aspirin for patients taking warfarin.

Acetazolamide
Generic term for Diamox, carbonic anhydrase inhibitor, used to treat edema.

Acetylcholine
This neurotransmitter at the end of a neuron innervates muscle.

Acetylcholinesterase
The cholinesterases that hydrolyze acetylcholine to acetate and choline within the central nervous system. Acetylcholinesterase inhibitor, (AChE). This is a group of drugs used to control myasthenia gravis.

Acromegaly
The term used to describe excessive growth after puberty.

ACTH
Commonly used abbreviation for adrenocorticotropic hormone.

Actifed
A commonly used drug for rhinitis, generic name of triprolidine/pseudoephedrine.

Acyclovir
This drug is administered in the treatment of genital herpes simplex.

Addiction
A psychologic and physical dependence upon a substance beyond normal voluntary control.

Addison   With this disease, there is a deficit of both cortisol and mineralocorticoid aldosterone.

Additive   When two drugs with similar action are administered, the drug interaction is called an additive effect.

Adenosine   This drug is the first-line choice to treat PSVT.

ADH   Commonly used abbreviation for antidiuretic hormone.

ADHD   Attention deficit/hyperactivity disorder.

Adjuvant   Medications that have been developed for other purposes and later found to be effective for pain relief in neuropathy are known as adjuvant analgesics.

ADL   The most commonly used abbreviation for "activities of daily living."

Adrenergic   This system is also called the sympathetic nervous system. Coreg (carvedilol) is an example of an adrenergic blocker.

Adsorbants   These agents act by coating the wall of the GI tract and adsorbing bacterial or toxins.

Adverse   This type of drug reaction is an undesirable drug effect that ranges from mild-to-severe effects. This type of reaction is more severe than side effects.

Afferent   Sensory neurons are also referred to as afferent neurons.

Afterload   The term used to describe reduced peripheral vascular resistance.

Aggregation   Clumping together of platelets to form a clot.

Agonist   A drug capable of combining with receptors to initiate drug actions; it possesses affinity and intrinsic activity. Opioid analgesics are called opioid agonists.

AHFS   An excellent drug information reference that provides accurate and complete drug information on nearly all US prescription drugs.

Akathisia   A syndrome characterized by an inability to remain in a sitting posture, with motor restlessness and a feeling of muscular quivering; may appear as a side effect of antipsychotic and neuroleptic medication.

Albuterol   This beta-adrenergic bronchodilator is used to reverse bronchoconstriction in anaphylactic shock.

Alcohol   One ounce of this substance twice a week may increase the risk of spontaneous abortion and may be responsible for FAS. The patient should not drink this when taking metronidazole.

Aliphatic   This phenothiazine produces a strong sedative effect and decreased blood pressure.

Aliskiren   Trade name of Tekturna. It binds with renin, causes reduction of angiotensin I and II.

Alkylating   These agents cause cross-linking of DNA strands and abnormal base pairing to prevent cells from dividing.

Aloe   This herbal supplement is not recommended during lactation.

Alopecia   Hair loss.

Alprazolam   Xanax. Used for alleviating anxiety that may cause sleeplessness.

Alteplase   This thrombolytic promotes conversion of plasminogen to plasmin.

Alveoli   Lung compliance is the lung volume based on the unit of pressure in the alveoli.

Alzheimer   This disease is an incurable dementia illness characterized by chronic, progressive neurodegenerative conditions with marked cognitive dysfunction.

Amiodarone   This agent is especially good for patients with impaired heart function who have atrial and ventricular dysrhythmias.

Amitriptyline   The generic term for Elavil. Antidepressant.

Amlodipine   The generic term for Norvasc, a calcium channel blocker.

Amoxicillin   This drug is an example of a low protein-bound drug.

Amphetamines   These stimulate the release of neurotransmitters from the brain and sympathetic nervous system.

Amphotericin   This polyene antifungal drug is used for treating severe system infection.

Ampule   A glass container with a tapered neck for snapping open and used only once.

Anabolic   These type of steroids are synthetic derivatives of testosterone developed to maximize anabolic effects of androgens.

Analeptics   These CNS stimulants mostly affect the brainstem and spinal cord but also affect the cerebral cortex.

Anaphylactic   Shock. An allergic response of the most serious type.

Androgen   Male hormone that promotes regression of tumors.

Anesthetic   A compound that reversibly depresses neuronal function, producing loss of ability to perceive pain and/or other sensations.

Angiogenesis   A physiologic process of new capillary formation from existing blood vessels.

Anion   Negative charge.

Anorexiants   Appetite suppressants.

Anoxia   Absence of oxygen.

ANS   Commonly used abbreviation for Autonomic nervous system.

Antacids   These agents promote ulcer healing by neutralizing hydrochloric acid and reducing pepsin activity. Taking these agents can prevent absorption of tetracycline from the GI tract. These agents should not be taken with iron because they impair absorption.

Antagonistic	When two drugs that have opposite effects are administered together, each drug cancels the effect of the other.
Antagonists	Adrenergic blockers.
Anthrax	May be used as a biologic weapon, highly lethal.
Antiandrogens	Androgen antagonists. They block the synthesis of androgens.
Antianginal	These drugs are used to treat angina pectoris.
Antibacterial	These agents are the treatment of choice for H. pylori.
Antibodies	Immunoglobulins.
Anticholinergics	Drugs that inhibit the actions of acetylcholine by occupying the acetylcholine receptors are called anticholinergics. This group of anti-ulcer drugs relieves pain by decreasing GI motility and secretions.
Anticoagulants	Group of drugs used to inhibit clot formation.
Anticonvulsants	Drugs used for epileptic seizures.
Antidepressants	Mood elevators.
Antidiarrheals	These agents treat diarrhea and decrease hypermotility.
Antidote	Synergistic drug effects act like an antidote.
Antiemetic	Another term used for antivomiting agents. An agent that prevents or relieves nausea and vomiting.
Antiflatulents	These agents are used to decrease excess gas in the stomach.
Antigen	Any substance that induces a state of sensitivity and/or immune response after a latent period.
Antihistamines	Drugs having an action antagonistic to that of histamine on either H1 or H2 receptors.
Antihypertensive	Diuretics have this effect because they promote sodium and water loss.

Antimetabolites	These resemble natural metabolites which recycle and breakdown organic compounds.
Antimicrobials	Antibacterials. Substances that inhibit bacterial growth or kill bacteria and other microorganisms.
Antimicrobials	These are used when infection develops from retained mucous secretions.
Antimycotic	Also called antifungal, these are drugs used to treat fungal infections.
Antiplatelets	This group of drugs is used to prevent thrombosis in the arteries by suppressing platelet aggregation.
Antiprotozoals	This group of drugs act by disrupting mitochondrial electron transport and inhibiting DNA synthesis.
Antipsychotics	Neuroleptics or psychotropics.
Antiretroviral	These types of medications are designed to slow or inhibit the HIV-related enzymes.
Antitumor	These type of antibiotics inhibit protein and RNA synthesis and bind DNA, causing fragmentation.
Antitussives	These drugs act on the cough-control center in the medulla to suppress the cough reflex.
Anxiety	The GABA neurotransmitter is associated with the regulation of anxiety.
Anxiolytic	A drug in this category, when administered, helps to relieve muscle spasms.
Apoptosis	The term used to describe cell death.
Apothecary	This system of measurement is no longer included on any drug labels.
aPTT	Commonly used abbreviation for activated partial thromboplastin time, lab tests to detect deficiency in clotting.

Artane   A brand name for trihexyphenidyl. Used to decrease involuntary symptoms of parkinsonism.

Arteriosclerosis   The primary cause of peripheral arterial/vascular disease.

Aspirin   This mild analgesic can inhibit the initiation of labor and prolong labor through its effects on uterine contractility.

Assessment   The first phase of the nursing process.

Asthma   An inflammatory disorder of the airway walls associated with a varying amount of airway obstruction.

Ativan   A trade name for lorazepam.

Atorvastatin   Trade name of Lipitor. Its mode of action is to inhibit HMG-CoA reductase.

Atropine   This sulfate is indicated in the treatment of hemodynamically significant bradycardia. It is a preoperative medication used to reduce salivation, increase heart rate and dilate pupils. It inhibits acetylcholine.

Atrovent   Ipratropium bromide. Bronchodilator used to treat COPD.

Azathioprine   Imuran. May be used in conjunction with lower doses of prednisone.

B

Bacilli	These bacteria are elongated in shape.
Bactericidal	These agents kill bacteria.
Bacteriostatic	These agents inhibit the growth of bacteria. Sulfonamides are considered bacteriostatic because they inhibit bacterial synthesis of folic acid.
Barbiturate	A derivative of barbituric acid, including phenobarbital and others that act as CNS depressants and are used for their tranquilizing, hypnotic, and anti-seizure effects.
Beclomethasone	Beconase. Used to treat allergic rhinitis.
Belladonna	This anticholinergic tincture is used to treat peptic ulcer.
Benadryl	Trade name for diphenhydramine, a commonly used antihistamine.
Benzocaine	This agent may be sprayed onto the perineum to relieve pain.
Benzotropine	The generic term for Cogentin. Used to treat extrapyramidal symptoms.
Betamethasone	Trade name of Celestone. Corticosteroid. An injection given to mothers to prevent respiratory distress syndrome in preterm infants.
Betaxolol	The generic name for Betoptic. A selective beta blocker used to decrease elevated IOP.
Bethanechol	The principal use of this drug is to promote micturition.
Bevacizumab	The generic term for Avastin, an angiogenesis inhibitor.
Biguanide	This compound acts by decreasing hepatic production of glucose from stored glycogen.

Bioavailability — A subcategory of absorption, is the percentage of the administered drug dose that reaches systemic circulation.

Biologic — Sulfonamides are not classified as an antibiotic because they were not obtained from these substances.

Biotherapy — This type of therapy augments the natural ability of the immune system.

Biphasics — This combination type fixes the amount of estrogen throughout the cycle.

Bisacodyl — Trade name of Dulcolax, a stimulant, increases peristalsis by direct effect on smooth muscle of the intestine.

Bismuth — This adsorbent is given for the prevention of traveler's diarrhea.

Blepharitis — The term used to describe an infection of the margins of the eyelids.

Blindness — Patients taking amphotericin B should be aware of this sign or symptom.

Bolus — IV push.

Bone marrow — Immune system cells originate in bone marrow.

Bortezomib — The generic term for Velcade and is used in the treatment of multiple myeloma.

Bowman — This is the double-walled epithelial cup also called the glomerular capsule.

Bradycardia — Slowness of the heartbeat, usually defined (by convention) as a rate under 50 beats/min.

Bradykinesia — Slow movement.

Brand — Trade name, also known as the proprietary name, registered trademark.

Brethine — Terbutaline. Bronchodilator. Used to correct bronchospasms.

Bretylium — The generic term for Bretylol. It prolongs repolarization.

BRM	The commonly used abbreviation for biologic response modifiers which is class of pharmacologic agents used to enhance the body's immune system.
Bromocriptine	Trade name of Parlodel. This ovulatory stimulant normalizes prolactin levels.
Bronchial	This type of asthma is a COPD characterized by period of bronchospasm with wheezing.
Bronchiectasis	An abnormal dilation of the bronchi and bronchioles.
Bronchodilators	These agents cause an increase in the diameter of the bronchus or bronchial tubes.
Bronchospasm	Contraction of smooth muscle in the walls of the bronchi and bronchioles, causing narrowing of the lumen. An adverse reaction to pyridostigmine administration may cause this.
BSA	This is the abbreviation for the method considered the most accurate way to calculate the drug dose for infants, children and older adults.
Buccal	This is the name of the route used when placing the drug between the gum and the cheek.
Budesonide	The generic term for Rhinocort, an intranasal glucocorticoid with anti-inflammatory action.
Bumetanide	The generic term for Bumex, a high-ceiling, loop, diuretic.
Butabarbital	Butisol. Relieves anxiety and as a short-term hypnotic for insomnia.
Butyrophenone	This group of agents is part of the nonphenothiazine group.

C

Caffeine	An analeptic used for newborns with apnea to stimulate respiration. Excess consumption of this substance may be toxic to the embryo. Intake of this CNS stimulant should be avoided by patients receiving targeted therapy.
Calcitriol	Trade name is Rocaltrol. This drug is used to treat hypoparathyroidism and manage hypocalcemia in chronic renal failure.
Calcium	Vitamin D has a major role in regulating calcium. Verapamil belongs to this class of channel blockers.
cAMP	Abbreviation for cyclic adenosine monophosphate.
Candesartan	The generic name for Atacand. May be used for patients who do not respond to ACE inhibitors.
Candida	This yeast is resistant to penicillin-type antibiotics and a common cause of infection of the mucous membranes.
Canister	A box or container.
Cannabinoids	The active ingredients in marijuana, a treatment to alleviate nausea.
Cantharides	Also known as "Spanish Fly" has been reported to cause bladder and urethral irritation and possible permanent penile damage.
Canthus	This term is used to describe a corner of the eye.
Capsule	This dose form is typically a gelatin shell that contains a powder or pellet.
Cardinal	The five responses to tissue injury are called the Cardinal signs of inflammation.
Carisoprodol	This drug might be prescribed to treat spasticity following a spinal cord injury.

Carvedilol   Trade name of Coreg. It is an alpha-blocker; nonselective beta1 and beta2.

Catecholamines   Chemical structures of a substance that can produce a sympathomimetic response.

Cathartics   These agents are used to eliminate fecal matter.

Caudal   Used as a local anesthetic, this block is placed near the sacrum.

Cefaclor   Trade name: Ceclor. This agent is a second-generation cephalosporin.

Cefdinir   The generic term for Omnicef.

Cephalexin   The generic term for Keflex.

Cephalosporins   Beta-lactam structure. They inhibit the bacterial enzyme necessary for cell wall synthesis.

Cerumen   Another term for earwax.

Cetuximab   The generic term for Erbitux used in the treatment of metastatic colorectal cancer.

Chalazion   An infection of the meiobomian glands causing blockage of the ducts.

Chimeric   Three types of engineered monoclonal antibodies include humanized, fully human antibodies and chimeric.

Chlamydia   This bacterial pathogen is transmitted predominately through sexual contact. Sulfonamides are most effective agains *Escherichia coli* and Chlamydia.

Chlorothiazide   This short-acting thiazide is used for peripheral edema. Its trade name is Diuril.

Cholinergic   Relating to nerve cells or fibers that employ acetylcholine as their neurotransmitter. An acute exacerbation of symptoms, cholinergic crisis.

Cholinesterase   One of a family of enzymes capable of catalyzing the hydrolysis of acylcholines and a few other compounds. Indirect-acting cholinergic drugs inhibit the action of this enzyme.

Chronotropic   This negative action decreases heart rate.

Chrysotherapy   Gold drug therapy.

Chylomicrons   These are large lipid droplets of reprocessed lipid synthesized and contain triacylglycerols.

Cimetidine   The generic name for Tagamet, an H2 blocker, blocks about 70% of acid secretions for 4 hours.

Clomiphene   The generic name for Clomid. An agent used as an ovulatory stimulant.

Clonic   This type of seizure is characterized by sustained muscle contraction.

Clonidine   Used primarily to treat hypertension, it regulates the release of norepinephrine by inhibiting its release.

Clopidogrel   The generic name for Plavix. An antiplatelet used for prevention of thromboembolism. It prevents ADP from binding with ADP platelet receptor.

Clozapine   The generic term for Clozaril.

Cluster   This type of headache is characterized by a severe unilateral nonthrobbing pain usually located around the eye.

CNS   Central nervous system.

Colchicine   This drug is the best choice when treating an acute gout attack.

Colitis   Inflammation of the colon. An adverse effect of taking lincosamides is pseudomembranous colitis.

Combivent   This is a trade name for the combination of ipratropium with albuterol used to increase bronchodilation.

Compliance   This is of utmost importance because discontinuing a drug before the course is completed may result in relapse.

COMT   Catechol-O-methyltransferase, outside the neuron. One of two enzymes that inactivate the metabolism of norepinephrine.

Constipation   An accumulation of hard fecal material in the large intestine.

COPD   Commonly used abbreviation for chronic obstructive pulmonary disease.

Cortex   The outer portion of an organ, such as the kidney, as distinguished from the inner, or medullary portion. The paired adrenal glands consist of the adrenal medulla and the adrenal cortex.

Corticotropin   This hormone stimulates the adrenal gland to secrete corticosteroids.

Cortisone   Drugs that may cause an elevated serum sodium level include cortisone preparations. Most of the wide variety of glucocorticoid drugs are frequently known as cortisone.

Coumadin   An agent that prevents blood clotting. The avoidance of large amounts of green, leafy vegetables is recommended for patients taking Coumadin.

COX   Second-generation NSAIDs. Selective COX inhibitors.

Creatinine   A component of urine and the final product of creatine catabolism. The creatinine clearance lab test is the most accurate way to determine renal function.

Cromolyn   This drug acts by inhibiting the release of histamine to prevent an asthma reaction. The generic name for Intal.

Cross   This is a type of sensitivity or allergy to one sulfonamide that may lead to sensitivity to another sulfonamide.

Cryotherapy   This therapy is used in the treatment of genital warts.

Cryptorchidism   The term used to describe undescended testis.

Crystalluria   A term used to describe crystals in the urine.

CTZ   Commonly used abbreviation for chemoreceptor trigger zone.

Cumulative   This effect occurs when the drug is metabolized or excreted more slowly than the rate at which it is being administered.

Cushing   This syndrome is a disorder resulting from increased adrenocortical secretion of cortisol.

Cyclopentolate   This drug may be used instead for patients sensitive to atropine sulfate.

Cyclophosphamide Cytoxan.

Cycloplegics   Agents that paralyzes the ciliary muscle and thus the power of accommodation.

Cytokines   These proteins regulate the intensity & duration of immune response.

Cytoprotectant   This type of drug, often given with high-dose cyclophosphamide, inactivates urotoxic metabolites.

Cytotoxic   Detrimental or destructive to cells. This type of therapy is often used to destroy cancer cells.

Cytoxan   Cyclophosphamide. This drug is helpful for patients with multiple sclerosis in the chronic progressive phase.

D

Danazol	This drug is a pituitary gonadotropin inhibitory agent
Decongestants	Assist in shrinking nasal mucous membranes and reduce fluid secretion.
Dehydration	Reduction of water content. One contraindication in the use of mannitol is dehydration.
Depolarization	Myocardial contraction.
DepoProvera	A long-acting injectable progestin, requires only one injection every 3 months.
Depression	A temporary mental state or chronic mental disorder characterized by feelings of sadness, loneliness, despair, low self-esteem, and self-reproach. The most common psychiatric problem affecting approximately 10%-20% of the population.
Dexamethasone	The generic name for Decadron. This agent has a rapid onset and shorter duration. Used as prenatal therapy for surfactant development.
Dextromethorphan	A non-narcotic antitussive that suppresses the cough center. It does not depress respiration.
Diagnosis	The determination of the nature of a disease, injury, or congenital defect. This is given as a result of analysis of assessment data. It aids in the development of a care plan.
Diazepam	This anxiolytic is used in the management of anxiety and alcohol withdrawal. Kava kava and valerian herbal supplements may potentiate central nervous system depression with the administration of this drug.
Dicloxacillin	Penicillinase-resistant penicillin
Digibind	This drug is the antidote for digitalis toxicity.

Digoxin	This glycoside is contraindicated in the case of ventricular dysrhythmia. It is used to treat heart failure, atrial tachycardia. An example of a drug that is low protein-bound.
Diltiazem	Generic term for Cardizem, a calcium channel blocker used for PSVT, atrial flutter/fibrillation.
Dimenhydrinate	The generic name for Dramamine, primarily used to prevent motion sickness.
Dimensional	Dimensional analysis. A calculation method known as units and conversions, decreases a number of steps required to calculate a drug dosage.
Diovan	This drug, an antihypertensive, may be easily confused with Dioval, an estrogen hormone.
Diphenoxylate	The generic name for Lomotil, combined with atropine, its mode of action is to inhibit gastric motility.
Disintegration	The breakdown of a tablet into smaller particles.
Distribution	The process by which a drug becomes available to body fluids and tissues. The pattern of occurrence of a substance within or between cells, tissues, organisms.
Diuresis	A term used to describe increased urine flow.
Divalproex	This drug is used to treat bipolar affective disorder for some patients in place of lithium.
DMARD	A commonly used abbreviation for "disease-modifying antirheumatic drug."
Dobutamine	Treats cardiac decompensation by enhancing myocardial contractility, stroke volume and cardiac output.

Documentation   The "Five-Plus-Five Rights" include the right: Client, drug, dose, assessment and documentation.

Docusate   This emollient comes in three forms: Calcium, potassium and sodium. Used as a stool softener.

Docusate   This stool softener is used as first-line treatment for constipation.

Dopamine   A neurotransmitter, a depletion of which causes parkinsonism. This sympathomimetic agent is often used to treat hypotension in shock not caused by hypovolemia. Antipsychotics act by blocking action of dopamine.

Dornase alfa   This drug is an enzyme that digests DNA in thick sputum secretions of patients with cystic fibrosis.

Doubling   The time it takes for the number of cells in a neoplasm to double, with shorter doubling times implying more rapid growth.

Doxapram   Used to treat respiratory depression caused by drug overdose.

Doxazosin   The generic name for Cardura. Used in the treatment of BPH.

Dram   A unit of weight: $1/8$ oz.; 60 gr, apothecaries' weight; $1/16$ oz., avoirdupois weight. The ounce and dram are more frequently used for measurement of fluid volume than for dry weights.

Dromotropic   This negative action decreases conduction of the heart cells.

Drop   A volume of liquid regarded as a unit of dosage, equivalent in the case of water to about 1 minim. Drop factor is the number of drops per mL.

Droperidol   This antiemetic is primarily used for prevention of nausea and vomiting during surgical procedures. (Inapsine).

DVT   Commonly used abbreviation for deep venous thrombosis.

Dyscrasias   Blood cell disorders.

Dyskinesia Impaired voluntary movement.

Dyspareunia Painful sexual intercourse.

Dysphagia Difficulty swallowing.

Dysphoria Major depression characterized by loss of interest in work and home, inability to complete tasks with deep depression.

Dyspnea Difficulty breathing.

Dysrhythmia Any deviation from the normal rate or pattern of the heartbeat.

Dystonia Facial grimacing, involuntary upward eye movement, muscle spasms of the tongue and face.

E

Echinacea Patients taking this herb may develop hepatotoxicity if given ketoconazole.

Echinocandins The action of this group is to inhibit biosynthesis of essential components of the fungal cell wall which interferes with growth and reproduction.

Eclampsia The term used to describe new-onset grand mal seizures in a patient with pre-eclampsia.

ECT Electroconvulsive therapy.

EEG A recording of the abnormal electric discharges of the cerebral cortex.

EGFR Commonly used abbreviation for epidermal growth factor/receptor.

Eldepryl   Selegiline. A MAOI used in the treatment of major depression.

Emesis   A term used to describe vomiting.

Emollients   Lubricants and stool softeners used to prevent constipation.

Emphysema   A condition of the lung characterized by increase beyond the normal in the size of air spaces distal to the terminal bronchiole.

Enalapril   The generic name for Vasotec. Used in hypertensive emergencies.

Endometriosis   The abnormal location of endometrial tissue outside the uterus in the pelvic cavity.

Endometritis   Intrauterine infection.

Enoxaparin   The generic name for Lovenox, one of four low-molecular weight heparins (LMWHs).

Entacapone   Comtan. A COMT inhibitor which increases concentration of levodopa.

Enteric   Hard-shell tablets must not be crushed because this type of coated medication may irritate the gastric mucosa.

Ephedra   This herb may increase the effect of theophylline and may cause toxicity.

Ephedrine   An example of a mixed-acting sympathomimetic which acts indirectly by stimulating the release of norepinephrine from the nerve terminals.

Epididymitis   A term used to describe an infection of the epididymis.

Epidural   The placement of this local anesthetic is in the outer covering of the spinal cord, or the dura mater.

Epilepticus   Rapid succession of epileptic seizures, status epilepticus.

Epinephrine   This drug is frequently used in emergencies to treat anaphylaxis. It is a potent inotropic that increases cardiac output.

Episiotomy   An incision to enlarge the vaginal opening.

Erectile	This dysfunction is characterized by persistent inability to attain or maintain a satisfactory erection.
Ergotamine	Not for prolonged use, but given to prevent or abort migraine attacks.
Erlotinib	The generic term for Tarceva, used in treatment for locally advanced non-small cell lung cancer.
ERT	Hormones for treating symptoms of menopause and decreasing risks of cardiovascular disease in postmenopausal women.
Erythromycin	This ointment is administered to the newborn immediately after birth.
Erythropoietin	Stimulates the formation of proerythroblasts & release of reticulocytes from bone marrow.
Esmolol	Used for treatment of SVT, atrial fibrillation and HTN.
Estazolam	ProSom. New benzodiazepine hypnotic for treatment of insomnia.
Estring	This is an elastomer ring inserted into the vagina where it releases estradiol for 3 months.
Eszopiclone	Lunesta. Treats insomnia.
Ethchlorvynol	Placidyl. Barbiturate-like drug used for sedation and sleep.
Ethnocultural	A combination of ethnic and cultural variables, perceptions.
Etoposide	This drug is an example of a topoisomerase II inhibitor. Used in treatment for small cell cancer of the lung.
Evaluation	This phase of the nursing process considers the effectiveness of teaching and attainment of goals.
Excipients	This term describes fillers and inert substances used in drug preparation.
Excretion	Four sequential processes of pharmacokinetics: Absorption, distribution, metabolism and excretion.

Exercise   This activity is an important aspect of nonpharmacologic method to reduce cholesterol.

Exfoliative   This type of dermatitis causes desquamation, scaling and itching of the skin.

Expectorants   These drugs loosen bronchial secretions so they can be eliminated by coughing.

Extravasation   The term used to describe that which passes out of a vessel into the tissues, said of blood, lymph, or urine.

Ezetimibe   The generic name for Zetia, a cholesterol-absorption inhibitor.

F

FAS   The most commonly used abbreviation for fetal alcohol syndrome.

Fasciculations   Involuntary muscle twitching.

FDA   The governing body empowered to monitor and regulate the manufacture and marketing of drugs.

Femcon   The first chewable birth control pill.

Femring   The first and only vaginal ERT to treat moderate-to-severe hot flashes, inserted into the upper vagina for 3 months.

Fenofibrate   The generic name for Tricor, used in treatment of type IV and V hyperlipidemia.

Fentanyl   The generic name for Duragesic.

Feverfew   Serotonin antagonist (herb) that relieves migraine headaches.

Fibrates   Another term for fibric acid.

Fibrinolysis The term used to describe fibrin breakdown.

Filgrastim The generic name for Neupogen. Its mode of action increases production of neutrophils.

Finasteride This steroid inhibits conversion of testosterone to dihydrotestosterone.

Flagyl A trade name for metronidazole.

Fluconazole This drug is part of the azole group and used to treat systemic fungal infection. This agent is given as primary therapy in the treatment of candidiasis.

Flumazenil Romazicon. Used in the management of benzodiazepine overdose.

Fluorouracil Antimetabolite. 5-FU.

Fluoxetine The generic term for Prozac.

Fluoxymesterone The generic name for Halotestin, a synthetic androgen, given for androgen deficiency.

Flutamide Antiandrogen. Eulexin. Men receiving this agent show elevations in plasma LH and testosterone.

Fluvastatin The generic name for Lescol, belongs to the group of statins.

Fosinopril The generic name for Monopril. Reduces peripheral resistance and improves cardiac output.

FSH The commonly used abbreviation for follicle-stimulating hormone.

Fungi These organisms are divided into yeasts and molds.

G

GABA   Gamma-aminobutyric acid.

Gamma   Interferon gamma enhances the oxidative metabolism of macrophages.

Ganglia   The nervous system is composed of all nerve tissues: brain, spinal cord, nerves, and ganglia.

Gardasil   This vaccine is indicated for girls and women ages 9 to 26 for prevention of cervical cancer and genital warts.

Gaviscon   A trade name for magnesium trisilicate, an antacid to relieve gastric disorders caused by hyperacidity.

GCSF   The commonly used abbreviation for granulocyte colong-stimulating factor.

Gelatin   An allergy to this substance requires that you hold administration of MMR.

Gemfibrozil   The generic name for Lopid, a bile-acid sequestrant.

Generic   The official, nonproprietary name for the drug.

GERD   The commonly used abbreviation for this disorder, an inflammation or erosion of the esophageal mucosa caused by reflux of the gastric mucosa.

Gestational   This type of HTN may occur without proteinuria after 20 gestational weeks.

Ginseng   This herb can inhibit the efficacy of furosemide. Taking this herb should be avoided during pregnancy as it is reported to decrease action of anticoagulants. This herb may decrease the effects of warfarin, thereby decreasing the INR. When this herb is taken with corticosteroids, central nervous system stimulation and insomnia may occur.

Glargine   Lantus. A long-acting insulin.

Glaucoma   Dopaminergics and anticholinergics are contraindicated in clients with glaucoma. Prostaglandin analogues are currently known to be effective in the treatment of this eye disorder.

Glipizide   Glucotrol. Second-generation oral antidiabetic.

Glucagon   This hormone is produced in the pancreas. It elevates blood sugar by stimulating glycogen break down.

Glucocorticoids   These members of the corticosteroid family are used to treat asthma.

Glycerin   This osmotic agent decreases volume of intraocular fluid to lower ocular tension.

Glycogenolysis   This term is used to describe the hydrolysis of glycogen to glucose.

Glycoprotein   G-CSF is a glycoprotein produced by monocytes and fibroblasts.

Glycosides   This group of drugs is used to correct atrial fibrillation/flutter. They inhibit the sodium-potassium pump.

GMB   A commonly used abbreviation for gastric mucosal barrier.

GMCSF   The commonly used abbreviation for granulocyte-macrophage colony stimulating factor.

GnRH   The commonly used abbreviation for gonadotropin-releasing hormone.

Goldenseal   Use of this herb is to be avoided in patients with glaucoma.

GoLYTELY   A commonly used evacuant given in preparation for GI examination.

Gonorrhea   Ceftriaxone is given as primary therapy in the treatment of this STD.

Gout   The "disease of kings."

Grain   In the apothecary system, the unit of weight is the grain.

Gram   In the metric system, this is the basic unit of measure for weight.

Granulocyte   A type of white blood cell that fights infection.

GTT   A commonly used abbreviation for drops.

Guaifenesin   Robitussin. Loosens bronchial secretions.

Gynecomastia   Breast swelling or soreness.

H

HAART   A commonly used abbreviation for highly active antiretroviral therapy.

Haloperidol   This drug alters the effects of dopamine by blocking dopamine receptors. Sedation and EPS may occur.

HCTZ   Commonly used abbreviation for hydrochlorothiazide.

HDL   This the abbreviation for the "friendly" lipoprotein.

HELLP   This syndrome is a severe sequela of preeclampsia and occurs in patients with gestational hypertension. It involves *h*emolysis, *e*levated *l*iver function, and *l*ow *p*latelets.

Hemorrhage   This is the major adverse effect of warfarin.

Hemorrheologic   Pentoxifylline (Trental) falls under the classification of this agent.

Henle   Nephron loop, extends into the medulla, then loops up to the cortex.

Heparin   A natural substance in the liver that prevents clot formation.

Heterocyclic   Atypical antidepressants, second-generation antidepressants, used for major depression, reactive depression and anxiety.

Pharmacology
Crossword Challenge
Glossary
Section XVIII

Hirsutism
Increased hair growth.

Histamine
The first mediator in the inflammatory process.

Homocysteine
Elevated levels of this have been associated with certain forms of heart disease.

Hordeolum
Local infection of eyelash follicles and glands on lid margins.

HRT
The most prevalent treatment for relief of vasomotor symptoms and vaginal dryness.

HTN
Commonly used abbreviation for hypertension.

Humalog
A rapid-acting insulin.

Hybridoma
This technology process uses mice to mass-produce monoclonal antibodies.

Hydantoin
These agents act by inhibiting sodium influx, stabilizing cell membranes.

Hydralazine
The generic name for Apresoline. An antihypertensive agent given for severe preeclampsia, causes arteriolar vasodilation.

Hydrochlorothiazide
The most frequent diuretic that is combined with an antihypertensive drug.

Hydrocodone
A narcotic antitussive. The generic name for Hycodan.

Hydrocortisone
This topical corticosteroid aerosol foam may relieve pain from hemorrhoids.

Hyperkalemia
Serum potassium level greater than 5.3 meq/L.

Hyperkinesia
Excessive motility, or muscular activity.

Hyperlipidemia
An excess of one or more lipids in the blood.

Hyperosmolar
Fluid which has more particles than water.

Hypertension   A common side effect for patient's taking Iressa.

Hyperuricemia   A term used to describe elevated serum uric acid level.

Hypochloremia   Decreased serum chloride level.

Hypoglycemic   Another term for oral antidiabetic drugs.

Hypokalemia   Low serum potassium level. This condition may occur with patients taking 50 mg of hydrochlorothiazide and digoxin 0.25 daily.

Hypomagnesemia   Low serum magnesium level.

Hypotension   This is a common side effect when taking drugs to treat BPH.

Hypothyroidism   A condition in which there is a deficiency of thyroid hormone.

Hypovolemic   This is the term used to describe shock resulting from loss of blood or fluid volume.

Hysterosalpingogram   The purpose of this exam is to evaluate fallopian tube patency.

I

Idarubicin   Idamycin. Antitumor antibiotic.

Idiopathic   Of unknown origin.

Immunoglobulins   Antibody proteins such as IgG and IgM. Elements of the immune response system.

Immunomodulators   These drugs treat moderate-to-severe rheumatoid arthritis by disrupting the inflammatory process.

Immunosuppressive   These agents are used to treat refractory rheumatory arthritis.

Implanon   This device is a single implant containing progestin and is an alternative method of contraceptive.

Indapamide   The generic term for Lozol, a long-acting thiazide and may be classified as a loop diuretic.

Infarction   An area of necrosis resulting from a sudden insufficiency of arterial or venous blood supply.

Infection   Caused by microorganisms and results in inflammation.

Infertility   The inability to conceive a child after 12 months of unprotected sexual intercourse.

Inflammation   A reaction to tissue injury caused by the release of chemical mediators.

Inhalation   The act of drawing in the breath; drawing a medicated vapor in with the breath; a solution of a drug or combination of drugs for administration as a nebulized mist intended to reach the respiratory tree.

Injection   Drugs given by this route involve only pharmacokinetic and pharmacodynamic phases.

Inotropic   This positive action increases myocardial contraction stroke volume.

Insomnia   The inability to fall asleep.

Integrase   This type of inhibitor blocks the insertion of HIV DNA into human DNA by attacking the enzyme that allows them to merge.

Interferons   A family of naturally occurring proteins.

Intoxication   State of being poisoned by a drug or other toxic substance.

Intradermal   This method of injection is usually used for skin testing to diagnose the cause of an allergy or the presence of a microorganism.

Intramuscular   The method of injection used for a more rapid absorption.

Intravenous   For outpatient surgery of short duration, this type of anesthetic might be the preferred form of anesthesia.

Iodine   Used in treatment of hyperthyroidism, to reduce the size and vascularity of the thyroid gland.

IOP   Commonly used abbreviation for intraocular pressure.

Ipecac   This syrup induces vomiting after poisoning.

Irinotecan   The generic term for Camptosar, used in treatment for advanced carcinoma of colon and rectum.

Iron   Ferrous sulfate, gluconate or fumarate.

Isoenzymes   The cytochrome P450 systems involved in drug metabolism.

Isoflurane   Forane. Not to be used as inhalation therapy during labor as it suppresses uterine contractions.

Isoproterenol   This beta-adrenergic drug is given to increase the heart rate.

Isordil   Isuprel, a beta-adrenergic, may be confused with this drug which is a nitrate vasodilator.

IUD   This device is inserted into the vagina and releases copper which interferes with sperm motility and fertilization.

IVPB   Commonly used abbreviation for IV piggyback.

J - K

Kaposi   This opportunistic sarcoma causes dark blue lesions and usually appears early in the course of HIV.

Kefauver Harris   Amendment. Legislation that increased controls on drug safety requiring adverse reactions be included on the label.

Keratitis   Corneal inflammation.

Ketoacidosis   A condition in which the body uses fatty acids (ketones) for energy.

Ketoconazole   This drug decreases the rate of drug metabolism which may increase toxicity for a patient on gefitinib.

Ketolides   A classification of antibiotics structurally related to macrolides.

Korsakoff   This is a name given to the type of psychosis producing a form of amnesia characterized by loss of short-term memory and inability to learn.

KVO   The abbreviation for keep vein open.

L

Labetalol   The generic name for Trandate. Used in cases of severe preeclampsia.

Lacrimal   This duct allows for passage of tears into the nose.

Lactation   Production and release of milk by mammary glands.

Lamivudine   Trade name Epivir. This drug is a member of the NRTI category.

Lamotrigine   Generic name for Lamictal.

Leucovorin   This "rescue" saves normal cells from the adverse reaction of MTX.

Levalbuterol   The generic term for Xopenex used in the treatment of acute bronchospasm.

Levophed   Norepinephrine. Used for shock, is a potent vasoconstrictor.

Levothyroxine The generic name for Synthroid. This agent is the drug of choice for replacement therapy in treatment of hypothyroidism.

Levsin Hyoscyamine. Treatment of peptic ulcer and IBS. Controls gastric secretion and spastic bladder.

Librax Combination of clidinium bromide and chlordiazepoxide, used to decrease anxiety and GI distress.

Licorice This herb antagonizes the effects of antihypertensive drugs.

Lidocaine An antidysrhythmic. This agent is considered an alternative to amiodarone. It exerts a local anesthetic effect on the heart.

Lidocaine Xylocaine. Introduced in 1948 as a nerve block, infiltration, epidural and spinal anesthesias.

Ligand Another term for a growth factor protein.

Linezolid This antibiotic is effective against MRSA, VRE and penicillin-resistant streptococci.

Lipids This term describes cholesterol, triglycerides and phospholipids.

Lipodystrophy Tissue atrophy or hypertrophy.

Liposomal This type of chemotherapy involves packaging of drugs inside synthetic fat globules.

Liter The basic unit of measure for volume in the metric system.

Lithium This drug was the first drug used to manage bipolar affective disorder.

Liver This organ is the primary site of metabolism.

Loading A large initial dose given when immediate drug response is desired.

Lopinavir Trade name Kaletra. Its mode of action is to inhibit HIV protease, rendering enzyme incapable of processing polyprotease precursors.

Loratidine   Commonly used drug for relief of allergic rhinitis and urticaria.

Lorazepam   Ativan. A benzodiazepine that acts by increasing the action of inhibitory neurotransmitter GABA to GABA receptor. Usually administered with an antiemetic such as metoclopramide. This drug may cause confusion and blurred vision.

Losartan   The generic name for Cozaar. It is a potent vasodilator and inhibits the binding of angiotensin II.

Luteal   PMS occurs in a repetitive regular pattern during this phase.

Lybrel   This is the first continuous-dose oral contraceptive pill to be FDA approved.

Lymphokine   Hormone-like peptide, released by activated lymphocytes, that mediates immune response.

Lypressin   Trade name is Diapid. This drug is used for prevention or control of diabetes insipidus caused by insufficient ADH.

M

Macrophages   The major phagocytic cells of the immune system.

Magnesium   This salt belongs to the class of osmotic saline stimulants, commonly known as Epsom.

Malfeasance   Giving the correct drug but by the wrong route that results in the patient's death.

Mannitol   This osmotic diuretic is used to treat cerebral edema and increased intracranial pressure, oliguria and to prevent acute renal failure.

MAO   Monoamine oxidase, inside the neuron, one of two enzymes that inactivates the metabolism of norepinephrine.

MAOI   Commonly used abbreviation for monoamine oxidase inhibitor.

Meclizine   The generic term for Antivert, is used to prevent nausea, vomiting and dizziness.

Meniscus   This is at the line of the desired dose.

Meperidine   The generic name for Demerol.

Mesolimbic   Brain reward system.

Metabolism   Another term for biotransformation.

Metaproterenol   The generic term for Alupent. Its mode of action is to relax smooth muscle of bronchi.

Metastasis   Spread of disease to other areas of the body.

Metaxalone   Skelaxin. Used in the treatment of acute, painful muscle spasticity.

Meter   The basic unit of linear measurement in the metric system.

Metformin   Glucophage. Nonsulfonylurea oral antidiabetic.

Methergine   This agent is prescribed for a patient with postpartum hemorrhage.

Methimazole   Trade name is Tapazole. This does not inhibit peripheral conversion to T4 to T3 and is 10 times more potent than PTU.

Methyldopa   The generic name for Aldomet. Used for stage 1 to 3 hypertension. Long acting. May be used alone or in combination.

Metoclopramide   The generic name for Reglan. Blocks dopamine receptors and is helpful in controlling nausea and vomiting.

Metoprolol   The generic name for Lopressor. Its mode of action is to promote blood pressure reduction via beta-blocking effect. This drug may cause a drug interaction in patients taking epinephrine.

Metric   All pharmaceuticals are manufactured using this system.

Metronidazole   The generic name for Flagyl. Used to treat H. pylori.

Midazolam   Versed. Used for induction of anesthesia and for endoscopic procedures.

Midodrine   ProAmatine. A drug used to treat symptomatic orthostatic hypotension.

Minipill   If this is taken more than 3 hours late, a back-up contraceptive should be used for 48 hours.

Miosis   Abnormal pupil constriction.

Miotics   These agents are used in open-angle glaucoma to lower the IOP.

Misfeasance   Negligence; giving the wrong drug or drug dose that results in the patient's death.

Misoprostol   The generic name for Cytotec, a prostaglandin analogue.

Mitotane   The generic name for Lysodren. This is an antineoplastic agent that suppresses action of the adrenal gland. Used to treat Cushing syndrome.

Mitotic   These inhibitors are derived from natural products and block cell division at the M phase.

Modafinil   Provigil. Used in the treatment of narcolepsy.

Molindone   The generic term for Moban.

Monoclonal   These antibodies, produced in the lab, are designed to bind to specific antigens on the surface of cancer cells.

Monophasics   Most common type of combination product.

Pharmacology
Crossword Challenge
Glossary
Section XVIII

Montelukast	This is the generic term for Singulair, a bronchodilator which inhibits smooth muscle contraction.
Morphine	An extraction from opium, this drug is a potent opioid analgesic.
Motor	Efferent neurons.
mTOR	Commonly used abbreviation for mammalian target of rapamycin
MTX	Abbreviation for methotrexate.
Mucolytics	These act like detergents to liquefy/loosen thick mucus so it may be expectorated.
Multiforme	Erythematous macular, papular or vesicular eruption.
Multiple Sclerosis	Common demyelinating disorder of the central nervous system, causing patches of sclerosis (plaques) in the brain and spinal cord.
Mumps	This disease produces swelling of the salivary glands, fever and headache.
Muscarinic	This receptor stimulates smooth muscle and slows the heart rate.
Myasthenia Gravis	A disorder of neuromuscular transmission marked by fluctuating weakness and fatigue of certain voluntary muscles.
Mydriasis	Dilation of the pupils.
Mydriatic	An agent that dilates the pupil.
Myelosuppression	Suppression of bone marrow activity.
Myocardium	This is the term for heart muscle.
Myxedema	This is a severe condition of hypothyroidism in the adult with symptoms of lethargy, edema of the eyelids and face, thickened and dry skin.

N

Nadir The lowest value of formed blood cells.

Nadolol Corgard. Used in management of hypertension and angina pectoris.

Nafcillin The generic term for Nafcin. Highly effective against penicillin G-resistant *Staphylococcus aureus*. This drug is an example of a moderately highly protein-bound drug.

Naloxone This opiate antagonist reverses the effects of all opiate drugs.

NANDA The most commonly used abbreviation for North American Nursing Diagnosis Association.

Naratriptan Amerge. Given for acute migraines, causes vasoconstriction of cranial carotid arteries.

Narcolepsy This condition is characterized by falling asleep during normal waking activities such as driving a car or talking.

Natamycin Trade name: Natacyn Ophthalmic, used as an antifungal. May cause transient stinging.

Natriuresis This term is used to describe sodium loss in the urine.

Necrosis Death of tissue caused by disease or injury.

Neomycin Frequently used as a preoperative bowel antiseptic.

Neoplastic These agents are examples of drugs that do not cross the blood-brain barrier.

Neostigmine Prostigmin. A short-acting AChE inhibitor. Used to increase muscle strength in myasthenia gravis.

Nephrotoxicity Toxicity to the kidneys.

Neurohypophysis The posterior pituitary gland.

Neuroleptic   Any drug that modifies psychotic behavior and exerts an antipsychotic effect.

Neuron   Muscle spasms have various causes, including injury or motor neuron disorders.

Neuropathic   This type of pain is an unusual sensory disturbance often involving neural supersensitivity.

Niacin   A trade name for nicotinic acid where doses are 100 times higher than RDA to lower VLDL.

Nicotinic   This receptor affects skeletal muscles.

NIDDM   Commonly used abbreviation for non-insulin-dependent diabetes mellitus.

Nifedipine   The generic name for Procardia. For HTN and angina pectoris, a potent calcium channel blocker.

Nitrates   These antianginals cause generalized vascular and coronary vasodilation.

Nitroglycerin   The drug treatment of choice for angina pectoris. This is one of several drugs considered an organic nitrates.

Nitroprusside   This sodium is an IV agent used to reduce arterial blood pressure in hypertensive emergencies.

NNRTI   Abbreviation for nonnucleoside reverse transcriptase inhibitor.

Nociceptors   These are sensory pain receptors activated by noxious stimuli in peripheral tissues.

Nocturia   Purposeful urination at night, after waking from sleep. This condition is a common symptom of an enlarged prostate.

Nonfeasance   Omission; omitting a drug dose that results in the patient's death.

Nonpharmacologic   These methods should be tried initially for pain relief.

Norepinephrine This catecholamine hormone is released from the terminal nerve ending and stimulates the cell receptors to produce a response.

Norflex Trade name for orphenadrine.

NREM Nonrapid eye movement.

NSAID The most commonly used abbreviation for nonsteroid antiinflammatory drug. These analgesics require ongoing assessment for GI bleeding.

NuvaRing This device is 2 inches in diameter, inserted into the vagina and releases estrogen.

Nystagmus Constant, involuntary, cyclical movement of the eyeball.

Nystatin Mycostatin. Administered orally or topically to treat candidal infection.

O

Oligospermia A subnormal concentration of spermatozoa in the penile ejaculate.

Oliguria Marked decrease in urine output.

Omeprazole The generic name for Prilosec. A proton pump inhibitor used to treat H. Pylori.

Onset The time it takes to reach the minimum effective concentration after a drug is administered

Opiates These agents decrease intestinal motility and decrease peristalsis.

Opioids Patients who receive this agent for pain should be assessed for bowel function and respirations.

Opportunistic This pathogen is capable of causing disease only in a host whose resistance is lowered, e.g., by other diseases or by drugs.

Orchitis   This term describes an infection of the testicles.

Orphenadrine   Norflex. For parkinsonism, antihistamine with anticholinergic effects.

Orthostatic   This type of low blood pressure occurs when an individual assumes an upright position from a supine position. Orthostatic hypotension.

Osmolality   The concentration of a solution expressed in osmoles of solute particles per kilogram of soluent.

Osmosis   The net movement of a solvent, which is water in living systems, through a selectively permeable membrane.

Osmotics   These agents are generally used pre- and postoperatively to decrease vitreous humor volume.

OTC   Drugs that are attainable without a prescription.

Ototoxicity   Damage to the auditory or vestibular branch of cranial nerve VIII.

Oxandrolone   The generic name for Oxandrin. An anabolic steroid given for delayed growth/puberty.

Oxygen   This gaseous element can be classified as a drug because it can have good and bad effects based on amount and manner administered.

P

Palliative   This type of therapy is used to relieve symptoms associated with advanced disease.

Pantoprazole   The generic name for Protonix, a proton pump inhibitor, used for treatment of gastric ulcers.

Paraplegia   Paralysis of both lower extremities and generally, the lower trunk

Parathyroid	This hormone regulates calcium levels in the blood.
Parenteral	This term describes medications administered intradermally, subq, IM and IV.
Parkinsonism	A chronic neurologic disorder that affects the extrapyramidal motor tract.
Paroxetine	This drug is an example of an SSRI.
Pathogens	Disease-producing microorganisms.
Paxil	A trade name for paroxetine. May be used for treatment of OCD.
PB	Abbreviation for protein binding.
PCA	The most commonly used abbreviation for "patient-controlled analgesia." This pump is programmed to administer prescribed medication at patient demand, and continuously.
PDE	Commonly used abbreviation for phosphodiesterase. These inhibitors facilitate erections by enhancing blood flow to the penis.
Pegylation	The process of adding a polyethylene glycol molecule to another molecule.
Penicillinase	This enzyme produced by the microorganism is responsible for causing its penicillin resistance.
Pentobarbital	Nembutal. Used for sedation, sleep or preanesthetic.
Pepsin	A digestive enzyme, this is activated at a pH of 2, and can cause mucosal damage.
Perimetrium	This is the outer layer of the uterus.
Permethrin	This cream rinse is applied as primary therapy in treatment of pubic lice.
Petit	Absence seizure. It causes a brief loss of consciousness, fewer than three spike waves on the EEG, usually occurs in children, petit mal.
Pharmaceutic	The first phase of drug action.

Pharmacodynamic   This phase is the study of drug concentration and its effects on the body.

Pharmacokinetics   The study of the time course of drug absorption, distribution, metabolism and excretion.

Phentermine   Adipex. Given for appetite suppression.

Phenytoin   Dilantin.

Phytochemicals   A term used to describe plant-derived compounds.

Phytomedicine   Medicine derived from plants.

Phytonadione   This agent, vitamin K, should be administered prior to circumcision.

Pilocarpine   This drug is a direct-acting cholinergic that constricts the pupils. It is used to treat glaucoma.

Piperadine   This phenothiazine has a strong sedative effect, causes few EPS and has no antiemetic effects.

Piperazine   This phenothiazine produces a low sedative and strong antiemetic effect and may have little effect on blood pressure.

Placebo   A pharmacologically inert substance. A psychologic benefit from a compound that may not have the chemical structure of a drug effect is known as a placebo effect.

Plasmin   An enzyme which digests the fibrin matrix of clots.

PMS   This syndrome comprises a collection of varied physical, emotional and behavioral symptoms.

PNS   Commonly used abbreviation for peripheral nervous system.

Polydipsia   Increased thirst.

Polyphagia   Increased hunger.

Polypharmacy   Administration of many drugs together.

Polyuria   Increased urine output.

Potentiation   This occurs when an additional CNS depressant is taken with alcohol, increasing the effect.

Prazosin   The generic name for Minipress. Its mode of action is to dilate peripheral blood vessels via blocking alpha-adrenergic receptors. Used for management of mild-to-moderate hypertension.

Prednisone   Its mode of action is the suppression of inflammation and adrenal function. It is readily absorbed from the GI tract and excreted primarily in the urine

Preload   This term describes the amount of blood returning to the right ventricle.

Procainamide   This agent is used in the treatment of ventricular tachycardia and PVCs.

Procrit   A trade name for epoetin alfa.

Proleukin   This interleukin-2 is FDA-indicated for the treatment of metastatic renal cell carcinoma.

Prolixin   A trade name for fluphenazine.

Promethazine   This antiemetic, The generic name for Phenergan, blocks H1 receptor sites & inhibits chemoreceptor trigger zone.

Propofol   Diprivan. Used for induction of anesthesia. Short duration of action. May cause hypotension and respiratory depression.

Propranolol   The generic term for Inderal. Used for management of angina pectoris, MI, HBP, dysthythmias. It is a nonselective beta1 and beta2.

Prostaglandins   Chemical mediators. Causes vasodilation and relaxation of smooth muscle.

Protamine   An antidote for heparin.

Protease   This is one of the three types of inhibitors that make up the classification of drugs known as antiretroviral therapy.

Proteasome   These inhibitors are intracellular multienzyme complexes that degrade proteins.

Prothrombin   This lab test measures the time it takes blood to clot.

Protozoa   This pathogen causes *Trichomonas.*

Proventil   Trade name for albuterol.

Proximal   Osmotic, mercurial and CAI diuretics affect the proximal tubule.

PSVT   The commonly used abbreviation for paroxysmal supraventricular tachycardia.

Psychosis   A condition whereby there is a loss of contact with reality.

Psyllium   This bulk-forming laxative (Metamucil) acts by drawing water into the intestine.

PTK   The commonly used abbreviation for protein tyrosine kinase.

PTL   Most commonly used abbreviation for preterm labor.

Puerperium   The period from delivery until six weeks postpartum.

Pumps   Electronic intravenous regulators.

Pyridostigmine   Mestinon. Used in the treatment for myasthenia gravis.

Pyrosis   Another term used to describe heartburn.

Q

QD   According to the Joint Commission, this is not an acceptable abbreviation for ordering or documenting medications.

R

Raloxifene   The generic name for Evista. A selective estrogen receptor modifier that increases bone mineral density.

Ranitidine   The generic name for Zantac, a histamine blocker which inhibits gastric acid secretion.

Rasagiline   Azilect. Interferes with dopamine reuptake at synapses in the brain.

Recombinant   This type of DNA is the genetic engineering process that produces mass quantities of human protein.

REEDA   The acronym for redness, ecchymosis, edema, discharge and approximation.

REM   Rapid eye movement.

Renin   An enzyme that converts angiotensinogen to angiotensin. Alcohol increases these secretions causing the production of angiotension II.

Repolarization   The return of cell membrane potential to resting after depolarization.

Retrovirus   HIV is considered this type of virus.

Rhabdomyolysis   This adverse reaction may occur in patients taking statins.

Rhinorrhea   Watery nasal discharge.

Rhogam   Human D immunoglobulin.

Rifampin   An example of a drug that is highly protein-bound.

Ritalin   This drug is typically given to increase a child's attention span and cognitive performance.

Ritonavir   Trade name Norvir. This drug is a member of the NNRTI category.

Rituximab   The generic term for Rituxan and is used to treat relapsed, low-grade NHL.

Rosiglitazone   Avandia. Nonsulfonylurea oral antidiabetic.

Rosuvastatin   The generic name for Crestor. Antilipidemic which may cut LDL in half.

S

Saddle   This local anesthetic block is given at the lower end of the spinal column.

Saluretic   This term is used to describe loss of sodium and chloride.

Sargramostim   The generic term for Leukine, increases production of eosinophils, macrophages, monocytes and neutrophils.

Scabies   *Sarcoptes scabiei.* Permethrin is used in the treatment of this condition.

Secobarbital   Seconal. A short-acting drug that may cause one to awaken early in the morning.

Selegiline   Eldepryl. Inhibits the catabolic enzymes of dopamine.

Senna   The generic name for Senokot. Used as a stimulant laxative.

SERM   Commonly used abbreviation for selective estrogen receptor modulator.

Seroconversion   The acquisition of detectable levels of antibodies in the bloodstream.

Sertraline   Zoloft. The most commonly prescribed antidepressant.

Silvadene   A topical sulfonamide used to treat burns.

Simethicone   Gax-X. An agent used to relieve flatulence.

Sims

This position is recommended to relieve hemorrhoidal pain and increase venous return.

Sinemet

A trade name for carbidopa-levodopa, dopaminergic, relieves tremors and rigidity.

Sinusitis

An inflammation of the mucous membranes of one or more of the maxillary, frontal, ethmoid or sphenoid sinuses.

Somatostatin

This group of antidiarrheals is given for severe diarrhea resulting from metastatic carcinoid tumors.

Sorafenib

The generic term for Nexavar, used in the treatment of metastatic renal cell cancer.

Sotalol

Betapace. Used to treat life-threatening ventricular arrhythmias and chronic angina pectoris.

Spacers

These are devices used to enhance the delivery of medications from metered-dose inhalers.

Spironolactone

The generic term for Aldactone, a potassium-sparing diuretic.

SSRI

Selective serotonin reuptake inhibitor.

Statins

This group of drugs inhibits cholesterol synthesis in the liver and slightly decreases the concentration of HDL.

STDs

Infections that are transmitted during sexual contact.

Stimulate

Cholinergics stimulate the parasympathetic nervous system.

Stroke

Cerebral vascular accident.

Subcutaneous

This method is used to inject drugs into the fatty tissue for slower absorption.

Subjective

Symptoms verbalized by the patient are considered subjective data.

Sublingual

This route of administration involves placing the drug under the tongue for venous absorption.

Sucralfate

The generic name for Carafate, a pepsin inhibitor.

Sulfisoxazole

The generic term for Gantrisin, a short-acting sulfonamide.

Sumatriptan

Imitrex. Adverse reaction, life-threatening, may cause coronary artery vasospasm, MI, cardiac arrest.

Sunitinib

The generic term for Sutent, approved for advanced renal cell carcinoma.

Superinfection

Occurrence of a secondary infection when the flora of the body is disturbed.

Sympatholytics

Drugs that block the effects of the adrenergic neurotransmitter are called adrenergic sympatholytics.

Synergistic

This type of effect is a coordinated or correlated action of two or more structures, agents, or physiologic processes so that the combined action is greater than the sum of each acting separately.

Synthesis

Azithromycin inhibits protein synthesis.

Syphilis

An acute and chronic infectious disease caused by the bacterium Treponema pallidum and transmitted by direct contact, usually through sexual intercourse.

T

Tachycardia

Rapid heart beat.

Tachyphylaxis

Rapid decrease in response to a drug.

Tacrine

The generic name for Cognex. Used to improve memory in mild-to-moderate alzherimer's dementia.

Tadalafil The generic name for Cialis. Used in treatment of erectile dysfunction.

Tardive This type of dyskinesia is a serious adverse reaction occurring in clients who have taken a typical antipsychotic drug for more than a year.

TCA The commonly used abbreviation for tricyclic antidepressant.

Tegretol Trade name for carbamazepine, has been used in place of lithium for some patients.

Temporality The perspective of time, determines whether the patient stresses a past, present or future orientation

Teratogens These are substances that cause developmental abnormalities.

Terconazole An appropriate treatment for vaginal candidiasis.

Tetracyclines First broad-spectrum antibiotics effective against gram-positive and gram-negative bacteria.

Theophylline This drug relaxes the smooth muscles of the bronchi, used for bronchial asthma. The best medication for a patient with an acute bronchospasm. Given through an NG tube, may be used for newborns with apnea to stimulate respiration.

Thioridazine The generic name for Mellaril.

Thiourea These derivatives are the drugs of choice used to decrease thyroid hormone production.

Thrombocytopenia A decreased number of thrombocytes in the blood.

Thrombolytics This group of drugs convert plasminogen to plasmin which destroys the fibrin in the blood clot.

Thrombosis Formation of a clot in an arterial or venous vessel.

Thyrotoxicosis Another name for Graves disease.

Tinnitus — Ringing, whistling, roaring sounds in the ears. This adverse reaction is typically caused by taking aspirin.

TobraDex — This is a combination of tobramycin and dexamethasone used in the treatment of fungal or viral infections of the eye.

Tocolytic — This type of drug therapy is used to decrease uterine muscle contractions

Tolazamide — Tolinase. A first-generation intermediate-acting oral antidiabetic.

Tolazoline — The generic name for Priscoline. Used for neonatal pulmonary hypertension.

Tolbutamide — Orinase. A first-generation, short-acting oral antidiabetic.

Tolerance — A condition in which larger and larger doses of a drug are needed to reproduce the initial response.

Topoisomerase — These inhibitors are nuclear enzymes that alter the shape of DNA coils.

Toxicity — This term refers to the first adverse symptoms that occur at a particular dose.

Toxoid — Inactivated toxins.

tPA — The commonly used abbreviation for tissue plasminogen activator.

TPN — Total parenteral nutrition.

Tramadol — Ultram. Contraindicated in severe alcoholism or with use of opioids.

Tranquilizers — This group of antiulcer drugs reduces vagal stimulation and decreases anxiety.

Transdermal — A type of medication administration whereby the drug is stored in a patch which may be placed directly onto the skin.

Travoprost — The prostaglandin analogue more effective in African Americans than non-African Americans.

Triamterene — Maxzide is a combination of hydrochlorothiazide and triamterene.

Trifluridine   The generic name for Viroptic, an antiinfective, used in the treatment of herpetic ophthalmic infections.

Triglycerides   Lipids are composed of cholesterol, phospholipids and triglycerides.

Triiodothyronine   Secreted by the thyroid gland. It regulates protein synthesis to stimulate mitochondrial oxidation.

Trimethoprim   This antibacterial agent interferes with bacterial folic acid synthesis just as sulfonamides do.

Triptans   These drugs treat migraine attacks.

Trough   The lowest plasma concentration of a drug, drawn before next dose is given.

Tuberculin   This syringe is a 1-mL syringe with markings in tenths and hundredths.

Typhoid   Salmonella enterica typhi.

U

URI   Upper respiratory infection. The common cold is the most prevalent type of upper respiratory infection.

Uricosurics   These drugs increase the rate of uric acid excretion by inhibiting its reabsorption.

Urinary   Bethanechol is a drug used to treat urinary retention

Urticaria   Hives.

Uveitis   Infection of the vascular layer of the eye.

V

Varicella Trade name Varivax. Used in the prevention of chickenpox.

VEGF This is the most important ligand involved in angiogenesis.

Ventilation This is the phase in which oxygen passes through the airways.

Vfend Trade name for voriconazole.

Vial A small glass container with a self-sealing rubber top.

Vinca This alkaloid is extracted from the periwinkle plant.

Vincristine Oncovin. Mitotic inhibitor. Affects cells in the M phase.

Virilization A term used to describe growth of facial hair and vocal huskiness.

VLDL The commonly used abbreviation for very low-density lipoprotein.

Vytorin This is a trade name for the combination of ezetimibe and simvastatin. Decreases absorption of cholesterol in the small intestine.

W-X-Y-Z

Warfarin Its trade name is Coumadin. This drug is an example of a first-pass effect drug.

Wheal This term describes a blister or a bleb.

Yasmin
This is the first oral contraceptive with progestin to reduce water retention.

Yohimbine
This natural product has been used with positive effects when taken to improve erections.

Zidovudine
The generic name for AZT. Its mode of action inhibits viral enzyme reverse transcriptase.

Zolpidem
The generic name for Ambien. Used for insomnia, this drug is classified as a nonbenzodiazepine.

Zosyn
Used to treat severe appendicitis, skin infections and pneumonia (piperacillin/tazobactam).

Zyloprim
This is not an antiinflammatory. It inhibits the final steps of uric acid biosynthesis. Used as a prophylactic to prevent gout.

Zyprexa
This drug is approved to treat acute mania.

Zyrtec
Trade name for cetirizine.

www.ingramcontent.com/pod-product-compliance
Lightning Source LLC
Chambersburg PA
CBHW081440170526
45166CB00008B/2264